Swag
PRESENTS

THE FLEXIBLE GOLFER

KYM COCO
M.A., RYT-500

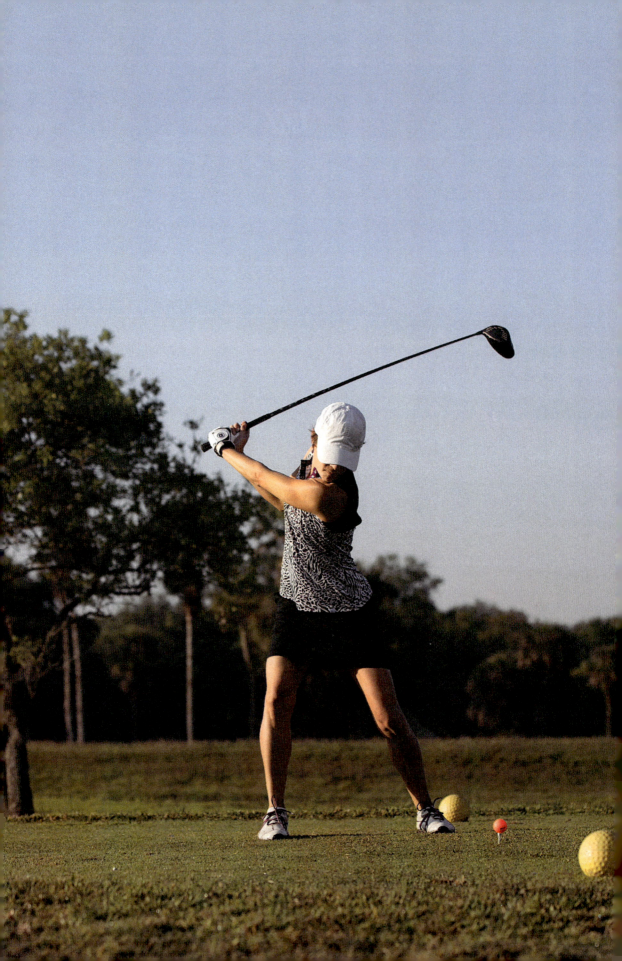

THE FLEXIBLE GOLFER

A guide to BALANCE your body,
FOCUS your mind, and IMPROVE your golf game

Kym Coco

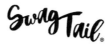

This book is written as a source of information only. The information contained in this book should by no means be considered a substitute for the advice of a qualified medical professional, who should always be consulted before beginning a new exercise or health program. All efforts have been made to ensure the accuracy of the information contained in this book as of the date published. The author, publisher, and contributors expressly disclaim responsibility for any adverse effects arising from the use or application of the information contained herein.

THE FLEXIBLE GOLFER: A GUIDE TO BALANCE YOUR BODY, FOCUS YOUR MIND, AND IMPROVE YOUR GOLF GAME

First edition

Contents Copyright © 2021 Swagtail, LLC. All rights reserved.

The Flexible Golfer © 2019 Swagtail, LLC. All rights reserved.

Golf Photography by Jina Morgese of Ember and Earth Photography

Content Design by Danielle Alling

Published by Swagtail, LLC

For more information, visit www.TheFlexibleGolfer.com

To my husband Steve, for the spark to start the game,

To my first coach Jennelle, for the skills to play well,

To my friend Diana, for the inspiration to play until my very last breath.

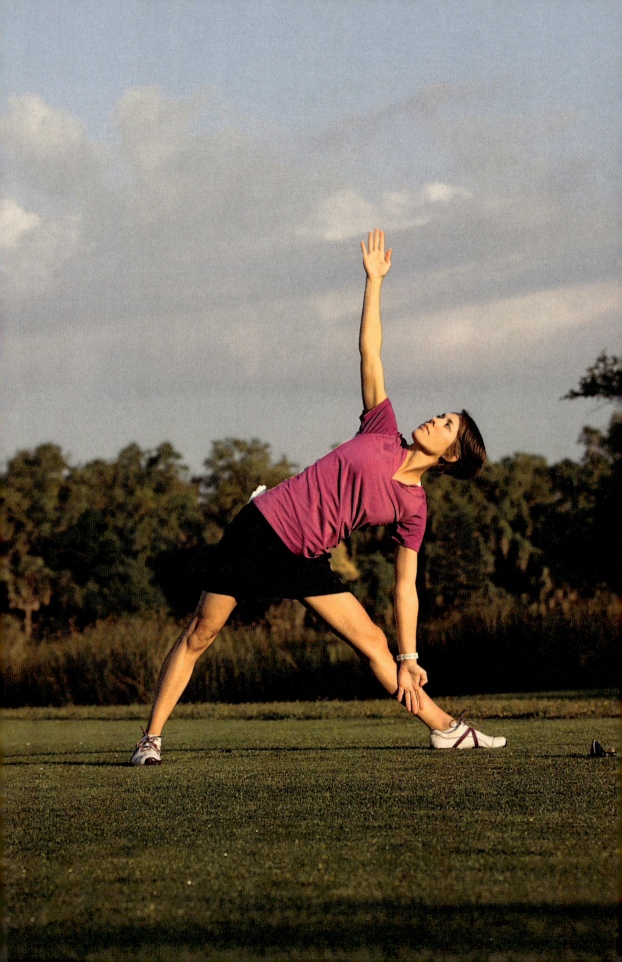

Contents

Author's Note   viii

INTRODUCTION   This Thing Called Yoga   1

WEEK 1   Discover the Golf-Body in Motion   27

WEEK 2   Flex the Muscles of Your Mind   49

WEEK 3   Develop a Pre-Round Routine   69

WEEK 4   Conserve Energy on the Course   91

WEEK 5   Post-Round Recovery   111

WEEK 6   Stay Golf-Ready All Year Long   143

CONCLUSION   Putting it Together   179

Next Steps   187
Acknowledgements   189
Resources   190
Index   194

Author's Note

The idea for this book began, like many great golf stories, with a memorable day on the golf course. I was in Santa Cruz, California for an advanced yoga teacher training program. Halfway through the 3-week intensive, I needed a break. I longed to trade the bamboo floor of the studio for a freshly-cut fairway. So I booked the only tee time available on such short notice—a 7:20 a.m. for the following morning.

I awoke in the dark to the loud bellow of the foghorn. Then after a quick stop at the local coffee shop for a hot latte and almond croissant, I started the hour trek south to the Monterey peninsula. As if on cue, the sun rays pierced through the gray mist just as I arrived at the course. I knew the day would be as beautiful as the forecasters predicted.

By hole 5, I found my groove. Oh how I had missed the grip of a club in my hand. My enthusiasm to play was only rivaled by the stunning views. The teal ocean lulled gracefully. Seagulls squawked as they circled the windless sky. The salty air filled my nostrils with each breath.

After a perfect drive on hole 13, my ball sat mid-fairway, 107 yards from the pin. I could only make out the tip of the flag, not because the fog obscured my view, but because of a rolling sand dune now covered in Poa annua grass.

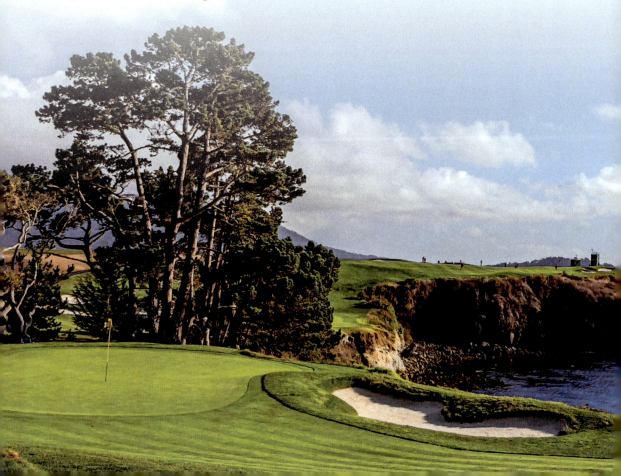

I grabbed my 8 iron—no sense in letting the dense, cool air prevent me from reaching my target. Then, ping! That sweet sound of solid contact that follows a smooth swing.

The ball soared high and straight toward the center of the green. It looked good. It looked better than good—it looked incredible. Suddenly, a cheer erupted from my playing partner, who had walked forward to check the results of his monster drive. Even the threesome on the elevated tee box ahead hollered, too. My ball had rolled right into the hole.

My first eagle landed unexpectedly. I didn't get the satisfaction of seeing it with my own eyes, but I didn't care. The resulting elation was the same.

If you're reading this book, you've probably experienced moments like these. Maybe it was a 40-foot putt that dropped (even when you just aspired to get it near the hole) or it could have been a hot streak that sent your spirits soaring.

These highlights reignite your passion for golf. They alter your perspective of what's possible in your own game and they fuel a desire to reach that potential regularly.

You see, the best part of my round that summer day in California wasn't the record-breaking number I posted on my scorecard. It was the realization that all the mental and physical training I had done on the yoga mat, and all the lessons I learned from the practice, had established my foundation for success on the golf course.

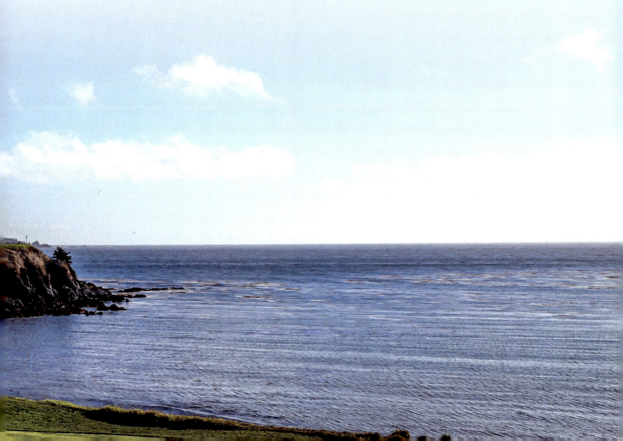

I'll share these specific techniques with you throughout this book.

I will teach you how to increase your physical strength, flexibility, and control. I'll cover how to conserve your energy and focus on what matters. Most importantly, I'll reveal how you can seamlessly integrate the body and mind in ways that create a more vibrant life experience.

It's this harmony we seek in golf.

Of course we prepare and refine our skills in advance. We analyze the game. We mentally rehearse our performance and enlist concentration to make strides in our abilities. Then, as we step up to the ball, we must let go of the mental flurry. We must release expectations, be present, and trust our swing.

When we do this, magic moments happen on the course. These experiences are often the goal—an endpoint to achieve. Yet they are just the beginning.

So if you're ready to push open the door of possibilities and uplevel your health, game, and life, turn the page and become a flexible golfer!

How to Approach This Book

While you might be in a rush to explore the actual yoga exercises in this program, I've found that lasting change occurs when golfers understand the root causes of their imbalance and the methodology behind a yoga practice. It also helps to have a clear direction in which to apply the information from this book.

That's why I define this thing called yoga first. I'll reveal the myths around yoga that prevent people from using it as a tool to enhance their game and the tips you'll need to know to start a practice of your own. Like golf, it's essential to understand the fundamentals. Then, week by week, we'll add a new element of yoga to improve your golf game.

In week 1, we dissect the golf swing. You'll learn which areas of the body require strength and which require mobility in order to prevent injury. I don't want you to end up like my friend, Derek, who spent the entire winter indoors, tore a rotator cuff muscle the first week of spring play, then missed the entire summer season. In addition to staying healthy, you can use this anatomical knowledge to optimize the coordination and consistency of your swing.

Week 2 transitions from the physical benefits of yoga to the mental ones. You'll discover how to flex the muscles of your mind, break negative patterns, and instill new habits that support your goals.

In week 3, we unearth yoga techniques you can use before each round to warm-up efficiently. This includes specific postures that prepare the body for the powerful golf swing. We also address how you can engage the mind and boost your energy, without burning out before hitting the first tee box.

Week 4 then becomes the path to sustain that energy throughout your round. You'll learn how to incorporate the breath to stay calm. You'll also master the use of your senses to remain focused on your game and keep distractions at bay. This is especially important when your playing partner is in the middle of their own downward spiral or you witness a bobcat leap from the bushes to attack the fawn running across the fairway. (Yeah, that really happened during my first season as a golfer!)

During week 5, you will learn the value of recovery post play. Not the cold beer and burger kind of wind-down that you find at the 19th hole, although that can be enjoyable, too. Instead, the activities this week use yoga postures and breathing techniques to restore your nervous system. This might not seem as sexy as the power you develop for a drive, but the long-term effects on your health, and the capacity to play well, are extraordinary.

In our last week together, week 6, you'll discover the best ways to incorporate yoga between rounds of golf. This builds an ongoing foundation from which to play with strength, stamina, and concentration.

All of this material is interactive. You'll gain new knowledge each week and I invite you to implement what you've learned at home (and on the golf course).

It's not meant to be overwhelming, though.

One of my favorite aspects of yoga—and a principle I frequently revisit throughout this book—is that simple changes can lead to the greatest benefits. The small habits you employ now can have the biggest impact on your golf game.

Ideally, you will plan a start date and work through this material sequentially. Yet if you travel a lot or have upcoming plans that could interfere, don't wait to get started. The perfect time might never appear. Just look for the best openings in your schedule. Set dates with yourself to learn and commit to the process.

There are also downloadable worksheets and yoga classes available at TheFlexibleGolfer.com/free to make this easier as you go.

Above all else, have fun! A playful attitude on the course, and the yoga mat, makes each experience far more enjoyable.

You can't see me now, but I'm smiling as I write this. I am so glad that you're here and I'm honored to guide you on this leg of your journey.

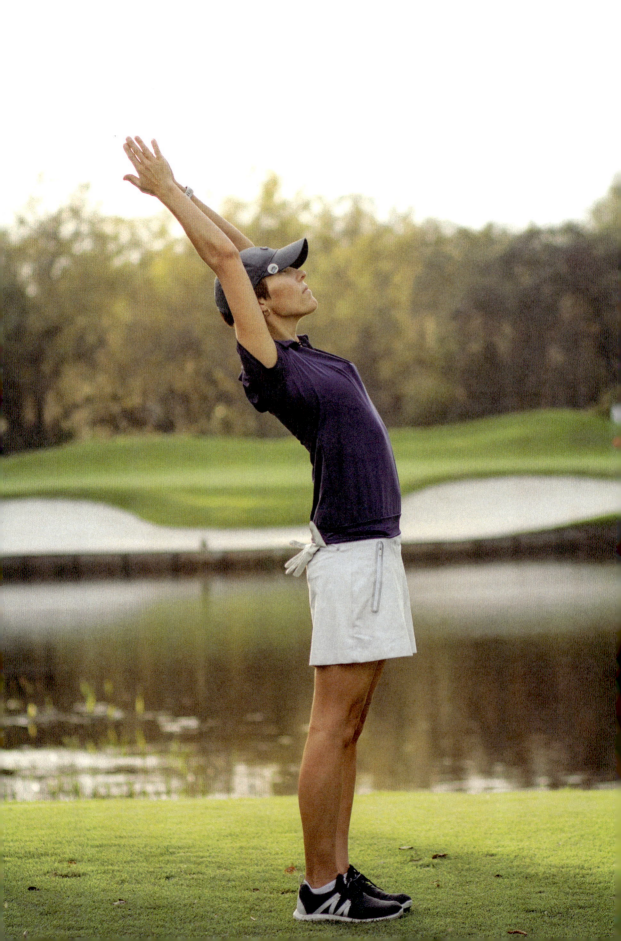

INTRODUCTION

This Thing Called Yoga

"If you understand WHAT you're doing and WHY you're doing it, the HOW gets much easier because you can assign meaning to what you're doing."

–Dr. Joe Dispenza

OVERVIEW

Yoga is an incredible tool to increase your physical prowess and mental focus on the golf course. To receive these benefits, you must first discover the foundation of the practice and how to use the techniques safely. You can then transfer your skills to your golf game with confidence.

Before we get into how you can use yoga to stabilize your hips ... Before we talk about how yoga can prevent low back pain ... Before we explore powerful yoga techniques to fine tune your focus and sink your tournament-winning putts ... I must reveal a secret.

The first time I tried yoga, I *hated* it.

It was my second year of college, and I was holding down two jobs just to put myself through school—the first of which was a personal training gig that had me seeing clients at 6 a.m. and the other was a Brown Forman promotion specialist (AKA Jack Daniel's girl) who worked late into the nights. Every waking hour in between was spent on studying to keep my Dean's list status.

If you detect my Type-A tendencies already, you're correct.

I took my first yoga class to garner academic credit while exercising. Yoga wasn't my first activity of choice, but it got me on the mat for the first time. Twice a week at 4 p.m. I would join the other students in our musty basketball gymnasium for an introductory yoga class.

Disappointingly, the experience was more like slamming on the brakes after traveling at 100 mph instead of reaching nirvana.

The movements were slow, and the teacher cued us in a low, monotone rhythm. I glared at her like you would at the back of the slow-playing foursome in front of you. Somehow I wished she'd get my telepathic message to speed things up so I could get on with the more exciting events in my life (like dinner with my new boyfriend).

My afternoon attendance soon became non-existent.

To be fair, I didn't do my research about yoga before taking this class. I'm the kind of person who will rip open a box as soon as it comes in the mail, pull out its contents, and try to figure out how the item works *prior* to reading the instructions. I like to figure things out with my hands.

So I had no idea yoga was more than an exercise regimen—although many styles of it today focus solely on moving the body. I didn't even realize that the physical postures came long after the origin of the practice thousands of years ago.

What is Yoga?

Yoga is ultimately a collection of techniques to harmonize body and mind. The word itself translates to union and yoga unites your focus with the present moment. It allows you to perceive a vast world beyond your body, roles, relationships, and circumstances to achieve a sense of effortlessness, freedom, and heightened awareness.

It's what athletes call *"the zone."* Each breathing method, body posture, and visualization technique within the practice is designed to help you get there.

Thankfully, a few years later, I was encouraged by a classmate to give yoga a second chance. This time I entered a small, local studio and was the youngest in the room by at least a decade. I quickly discovered that my youthfulnes didn't give me an advantage, and any star-athlete status from my past didn't cut it either.

I could only compensate for my inability on the mat with laughter. Loud. Uncontrollable. Room-stopping, belly-rolling laughter.

My postures *did not* look anything like those of the seasoned practitioners in the room, which I learned doesn't really matter in yoga anyway.

What got me hooked in that sweaty, dark studio was the challenge. This is probably what initiated my golf-obsession, too. Both require strength, stamina, finesse, and focus.

Both are awkward at first. Yet, with time, the unnatural becomes less so. The weird becomes second nature. And you're able to see tangible outcomes.

> "The most effective way to improve a golf game is to improve the quality of the body playing the sport. As players are in better control of their bodies, it becomes easier to improve the technical part of their game because now they have more movement options available."
>
> –Dr. Craig Davies[1]

As a result of starting a regular yoga practice, my stress levels declined. I slept better at night. My body weight normalized. My skin cleared up. I even had an inner sense of calm in spite of having absolutely no idea what job awaited me after graduation.

Research data[2] backs up my experience and shows that yoga leads to:
- Greater flexibility
- Better blood circulation
- Improved cardiac function
- Greater immunity
- More balanced moods
- Reduced pain levels
- Less irritability
- Lower heart and respiratory rates
- Less fatigue
- Less stress.

As for you, fellow golf-lover, yoga is a practice that can help keep your body safe and strong on the course. It also gives you the foundation from which to play well for many, many more years to come.

Here's how yoga gets you golf-ready:

Yoga Increases Mobility

Maybe you thought the first benefit of yoga would be increased flexibility. That's actually what most people think of when they hear about yoga. They envision Gumby or Stretch Armstrong or a crazy-talented gymnast. This is because yoga postures really do increase the length of your muscular tissue and improve joint range of motion.

However, flexibility is worthless without control.

That's where mobility steps in. Mobility is how you control your movements. Mobility gives you the power to deliberately move in more flexible ways.

This is especially important with regards to a powerful golf swing. Every time you strike the ball, most of your body's joints move through a large percentage of their maximum range of motion.

If you're overwhelmed by this anatomical terminology, I understand. I almost changed majors the first week of my anatomy class due to this fact. (Well, because of that and the burned-out professor with chalk-stained fingers who didn't make any effort to glamorize the subject.)

Since I want you to stick around, I'll simplify the anatomical lingo.

A joint is where two or more bones connect and these joints allow for motion.

Which joints of the body might you need to be healthy and mobile to create a powerful golf swing?

You guessed it—at the spine!

The spine consists of 33 individual bones, stacked one on top of the other, and contains multiple joints at each level. This spinal column provides the main support for your entire body, allowing you to stand upright, bend, and twist. It's also responsible for protecting the spinal cord from injury.

Each of these controlled spinal movements allows you to hit the golf ball better. Yogis, too, understand the value of a mobile spine. In fact, they go so far as to say that the quality of life is determined by the flexibility of the spine.

That's why yoga moves the spine in all functional directions. It also helps build strong and flexible muscles, ligaments, and tendons around the spine so that you can move it with more control. More control of your flexibility leads to better mobility, which is true on your yoga mat and the golf course.

> **NOTE:** As a golfer, you want maximum healthy movement at the spine to create a powerful golf swing.

Yoga Boosts Your Balance

A golf-ready body also requires balance. What makes golf unique when compared to many other sports is that the ground on which you play is unpredictable. The slope and firmness of the surface beneath you changes all the time.

One minute you could be playing on firm short grass with a downhill slope. The next, you're forced to hit out of soft sand with an uphill lie. This constant adjustment requires a significant amount of balance and coordination in the lower body to remain steady so that the spine can rotate into the correct position for your swing.

What you might not realize is that greater balance begins with the feet.

That's why yoga teaches you how to:
- Activate your feet properly
- Distribute weight evenly
- Transfer weight safely from one foot to the other when taking yoga postures on the mat (and in the various positions needed in your golf game)

- Decipher changes in the feet
- Use information from the feet to make better decisions

Basic exercises in week 1 will show you how to boost balance in your feet right away.

Balance = Harmony

Not only is balance known for keeping you upright when walking and swinging a golf club, balance also refers to a sense of inner harmony. In scientific terms, it's called equilibrium or homeostasis. You might know it as *"finding your center."*

> *"Balance is a moving target."*

Your body is working 24/7 to find internal balance. Yet daily activities can make that more challenging. What you consume and think about affects your physiology. So does the air quality and toxin levels of your environment. Even how you move on a regular basis impacts your equilibrium.

Take the golf swing, for example.

During any given round, you're continually swinging your club in one direction, with lots of power, for hours on end. This action creates an imbalance in the muscles just by the very nature of the swing.

Simple daily habits can also contribute to unevenness. You might repeatedly carry a bag or baby on one arm. Or maybe you sit behind a desk for hours at work. Even small tasks like brushing your teeth and hair with a dominant hand can fuel imbalances.

These asymmetrical actions might not cause a big problem today. However they can have devastating effects like unwanted pain, limited mobility, or overuse injuries in the future.

My client, Dan, knows this well. His career as a truck driver had him sitting for hours on end. He was also a dedicated weekend golfer. This combination led to chronic lower back discomfort. Instead of quitting the game, he wore a back brace to offset his weak core, tight hamstrings, and lumbar ache. Dan knew this was unsustainable, so he started a regular yoga practice with me. Within two years, he saw remarkable improvement. He was able to ditch the back brace and drop his handicap by 5 strokes.

This is just one example of how yoga restores equilibrium. You strengthen areas that are weak, or underutilized, and you stretch muscles that get tense or over-worked. Yoga highlights these imbalances so you can fix them and prevent them from getting worse over time.

Yoga Enhances Body Awareness

Another way yoga improves your golf game is with greater body awareness. This is known as proprioception (pro-pree-o-sep-shen), which is just a fancy way of saying that your body understands how it is moving in relation to other parts of itself and with the environment around you.[3]

Sensory organs, called mechanoreceptors, constantly collect data from your environment. These mechanoreceptors are located throughout your body, with an exceptionally high density in the feet. Once these sensory cells absorb information, they relay it to the brain via the connective tissue and nervous system.

In the broadest sense, a yoga practice heightens the awareness of your entire body. On a subtle level, yoga increases the accuracy of how that information is received. It also increases the speed at which that information is processed.

This translates directly to increased levels of coordination. All your body segments now work with greater efficiency to hit a golf ball. And you can do so with more efficiency and power than ever before.

Yoga Builds Strength and Power

Strength and power are two unlikely words to be paired with a yoga practice. Yet yoga is one of the best ways to build these elements in a golf-ready body. Let's look at strength first.

Strength refers to the amount of force a muscle group can produce. Just think about the strength required to hold your club up in space. Your core, back, shoulders, and arms all fight against gravity to get into proper position for your backswing. This can be a challenge for many new golfers. They experience muscular fatigue before hitting the turn because they can't sustain the needed strength to swing over time. That's called endurance.

Then power comes into play as you forcefully move your club into the downswing. Power involves strength; only it adds the variable of time into the equation. To put it simply, strength + speed = power.

Before you can understand how yoga increases strength and power, you must first learn some muscle anatomy. A muscle has two basic states—a resting state and a contracted state. When at rest, muscle fibers are long and they store energy for later use.

Muscles then shorten, or contract, upon neural impulses. This is the foundation of all body movements and you build strength in the muscles by exposing them to increased resistance over time.

With yoga, you build strength by progressively overloading your muscles. This makes them longer and larger with practice.

On the yoga mat, your own body weight is used as resistance. You fight gravity to keep your arms parallel to the floor or you press the ground away to stay steady in a plank position. As your strength improves, you can intensify the challenge on the yoga mat. Thanks to greater coordination and increased body awareness, you can do all these movements at greater speed, too. The strength you establish in yoga then transfers to the course to sustain your golf swing.

Get Rid of Unwanted Tension

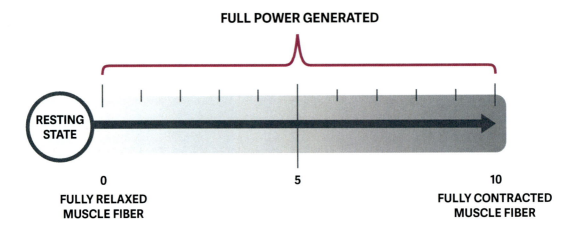

Yoga also trains your muscles into a fully rested state. The above diagram simplifies this concept. At zero, a muscle fiber is completely long and relaxed. At ten, it's short and contracted to its fullest capacity.

Yoga teaches muscle fibers to relax when not in use. From this elongated position you can then fully contract and gain maximum power from that muscle. The hypothetical value for this power output would be a 10 on the scale (10 - 0 = 10). This gives you more energy to move and the capacity to do so for longer periods of time. Think greater swing speeds and further distance with your golf shots.

Only most people don't let their muscles relax. Instead, the muscles remain in a state of chronic muscular tension, meaning that the fibers are using energy unnecessarily. They aren't storing any reserves for later, and when they go to contract, they generate less strength overall.

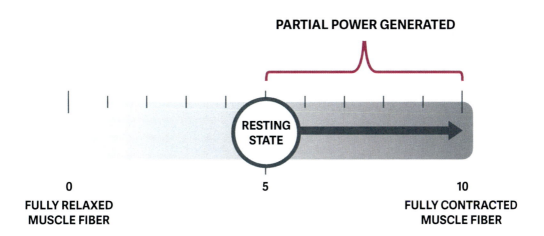

Said another way, the partially rested muscle might linger around the halfway mark on the scale. When recruited for use, the muscle can then only produce an output of 5 (10 - 5 = 5). This is far less than it could from a fully rested state. Because the muscle was also wasting energy in this middle ground, you might not be able to fully contract the muscle at all. And even if you could, the high output won't last for long. This muscular inefficiency can cause unwanted injuries and lead to more inconsistency as you fatigue during play.

That's why we use yoga postures throughout this book to develop the strength, endurance, and power you seek to stay golf-ready all year long!

Yoga Heightens Your Focus

It's true that all the physical benefits I just mentioned can significantly improve your golf game. Nevertheless, I've saved my favorite benefit for last. Yoga heightens your focus. It trains the mind to be present and work in harmony with your body.

Since the mind is the brain in action, it's important that you understand some basics about the brain.[4]

- The brain is a bioelectrical organ that accounts for 2% of your total body weight as an adult.
- The electrical activity that emanates from the brain is displayed in the form of brainwaves.

- Each brain wave pattern releases certain chemicals into the body.
- Slower brain waves are associated with staying calm and relaxed regardless of the external environment. We'll talk more about this on page 53.

The physical postures, breathing techniques, and visualization activities of yoga all train your mind into these slower brain wave patterns.

How does this help your golf game?

Imagine you're having a great round. Your swing is effortless and you (amazingly) keep hitting shots right where you want them to go. You are totally in the zone. Then, as you're about to post your lowest score of the season, you pull the ball directly into the large water hazard on hole 16. My gut-to-mouth response is often a four-letter word that you don't want the kids to overhear.

Regardless of what you say silently or aloud, that shot is now in the past. A trained mind can quickly let go of that mishap and refocus with precision. With greater focus, your upcoming hit can reach the target instead of triggering a domino effect of extra strokes on your scorecard.

Yoga Myths

Yoga can be categorized in many ways. It's a workout, training tool, or lifestyle. Many even refer to it as a spiritual path. Yoga has thousand-year-old roots and it's being modified on a daily basis. This can cause confusion about the practice. This confusion perpetuates the yoga myths you hear today and it also prevents many individuals, including golfers, from giving yoga a try.

A myth is a commonly held idea or belief not founded in the truth. Some common myths present in human history are that the Earth is flat, Earth is the center of the Universe, or fascia is an entirely useless aspect of the body. Not sure what fascia is? Get the details on page 119.

The common myths I hear about yoga are that it's a fitness trend or brainwashing cult. My favorite: yoga is something only flexible people do. I wouldn't have been admitted to my first class, nor would I still be practicing today, if that were actually true.

The beauty of yoga is that it's open to all ages, sizes, genders, races, and ability levels. The same benefits that ancient yogis received are now backed by scientific research. And the amazing access to information on the internet today helps you blend common sense with social proof to form your own opinion. That's likely one of the reasons this book is in your hands right now.

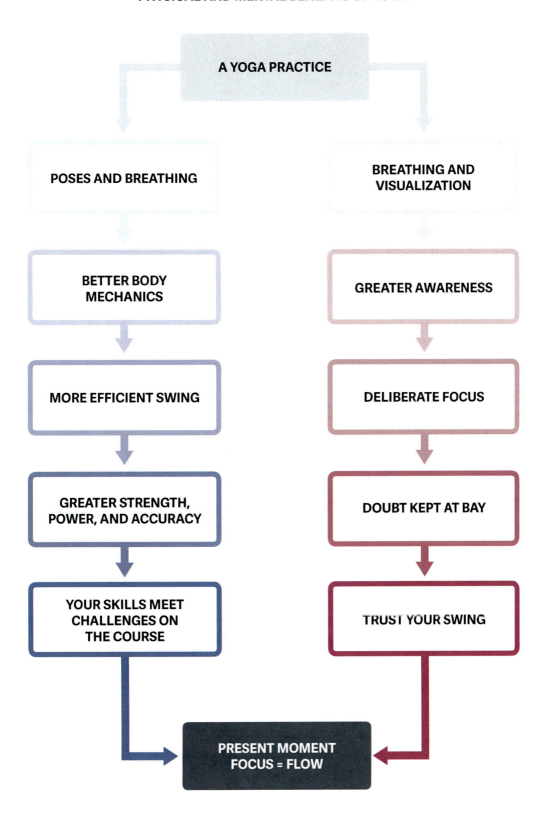

My hope is that by uncovering the common myths of yoga, any lingering doubts in your mind about the practice will be put to ease.

Myth: Yoga is a Religion

Yoga originated in India—the current home to 1.3 billion people, a majority of whom follow the Hindu tradition. Combine that fact with the chanting and mantras still used in modern-day yoga classes, and it's no wonder yoga is perceived as a religion.

But it's not!

From the beginning, yoga was a methodology designed to help people understand their infinite potential. Ancient yogis used it as a tool for self-realization. Said another way, yoga was designed to help you understand your inner world. It's a way to make peace with the unknowns in life, such as: Is this the right decision? Am I on my path? Does my life make a difference in the vast scope of the Universe?

If those are questions you're asking now, I, as a yoga teacher, don't have answers for you. Only the wise voice within you can answer these questions. Yoga simply helps you tap into your inner wisdom on a regular basis via movements, breathing techniques, and focused awareness.

In fact, the quiet rest at the end of a yoga class gives you space to listen. In this reflective time, you are given the ability to absorb the physical and mental changes made during your practice. Better still, the common motto that *"you're limitless"* actually takes hold in the body.

Many yoga students report feeling extremely peaceful or calm after class. They extend more grace to themselves and others, and they're more alert and composed.

> **TIP:** The unfamiliar language you hear in yoga is called Sanskrit. It's one of the oldest known languages in the world and it's not tied to any particular religion. I use Sanskrit words throughout this text for two reasons. First, I want you to be familiar with some yoga jargon should you venture into a yoga class. Second, many Sanskrit words don't translate well (or easily) into the English language.

In the past, religious domains only told of such transcendent experiences. Yet yoga doesn't come with religious dogma or a set of rules to awaken such states of consciousness. You don't have to practice any particular style, or attend a certain number of classes each week, to get results.

Yoga just requires the courage to look inward. And, because yoga is a way to honor the spiritual essence at the heart of humanity, it dovetails nicely into any religious philosophy you already have in place.

Myth: You Must be Flexible to Do Yoga

On the surface, yoga appears to many to be a set of calisthenic exercises to achieve greater physical fitness. I'm going to switch countries for a moment and introduce you to the Greek roots of calisthenics. *"Kalos"* means beauty and *"Stenos"* means strength.

It's no wonder that pictures of strong and beautiful yogis spread like wildfire on social media channels. Who doesn't like to look at a stunning gymnast upside-down on fingertips?

The problem is, those extremes are not relatable to a majority of the population (myself included). And those images fuel the myth that you must be flexible to practice yoga in the first place.

Flexibility isn't a requirement to start yoga; it's a byproduct of doing it.

Yoga is for every body, no matter what body you bring to the practice. You might be tall or short. You could be thick or thin. Young or old. Doesn't matter.

My husband often jokes that he's in shape. This is because round is a shape!

He doesn't have the stereotypical thin yoga body. He can't even come close to touching his toes. Due to a motorcycle accident in the 1990s, his chest is grafted on his shin and one butt cheek is shaped by silicon. I'll leave you to guess which one that is when you meet him.

Even he can do yoga.

Yoga didn't start with a physical emphasis thousands of years ago. And it's only part of the process still today. The end result is the same for anyone willing to give it a try; you become more flexible in body and mind from your practice.

Myth: Yoga is Too Easy

Our culture is obsessed with promoting the motto *"no pain, no gain"* especially in the realm of health. This might make some of the less physical forms of yoga—like Restorative, Yin, or Chair Yoga—seem too easy.

- Yin Yoga uses long holds at 50% capacity to elongate the connective tissue, tendons, and ligaments, which increases functionality and overall range of motion.
- Restorative Yoga also uses supportive, mild postures to reset the nervous system. This removes the unwanted side effects of stress such as inflammation, high blood pressure, and anxiety.
- Chair Yoga is a practice that skips poses on the floor and instead uses a chair to strengthen, elongate, and balance the body.

We'll tap into each of these styles in week 5 to help your body recover after a round of golf.

The subtle benefits that gentle yoga postures provide are undervalued. This continues the myth that yoga is too easy and causes many to overlook yoga as a beneficial training tool.

The truth is, yoga requires the body and mind to work together fully, present, and engaged in the moment. It's different than walking on a treadmill while watching TV or walking around the neighborhood while listening to your favorite podcast. Those activities can distract the mind while the body is in motion.

On the yoga mat, you link the body and mind with the breath. And when there is less movement of the body, it can be more challenging to rein in the mental chatter, which makes yoga much more challenging that it may appear on the surface.

Myth: Yoga is too Hard

Another myth is that yoga is too hard. It's often perceived as intimidating; full of postures that could never be accomplished, much less attempted. This myth discourages many from starting a yoga practice at all.

So if you think yoga is too difficult, I'll say it again: Yoga is a practice designed to meet you where you're at.

Yoga is not meant to force your body into any kind of pose. You're not meant to endure pain. Nor do you need to go deeper, faster, or harder in practice to receive benefits. In fact, the opposite is true. You want to adopt a yoga pose to fit your body—not fit your body into the pose.

Similarly, I'm not out on the course trying to swing like Tiger Woods. His clubs wouldn't fit me, and his shoes would be way too big. There are times, though, where I do harness my inner pro. I hold my head high, sashay with a little swagger, and even wear red on Sundays. Okay, red is not my color, so I wear purple instead. It's not the actual color that matters. It's the winning mentality on game day that does.

On the course, I recognize that I'm not Tiger, and I don't have to be. I can play my game and improve at my own pace. We can all recognize the challenges of golf and authentically rise to meet the various demands. The same is also true on the yoga mat. It's the magic of finding your own flow in both that keeps us coming back for more.

Myth: Yoga is a Fad

This myth follows the premise that yoga is just a new and trendy exercise program that will be replaced by the next gimmick any day now. The truth is yoga has been around for thousands of years as a way to integrate the various, complex layers of your life.

The word yoga in Sanskrit means "*union.*" It is a worldview designed to bring the body, mind, and spirit into harmony with one another. It's a way to balance the many facets of yourself. Ideally, it's a practical way in which your golf-loving nature can coexist with your passion for horses, gardening, or travel.

Yoga is a way to connect you with the very best version of yourself at any given moment. The practice ignites your potential. Physical postures shake off old, destructive patterns, and breathing techniques bring your focus into the present.

Yoga resources available today are fresh ways of communicating these timeless concepts. In this book, we're using yoga to improve your golf game. You'll soon discover, though, that the principles you learn here (and the benefits you will receive) extend far beyond the tee box, fairway, and greens.

Foundations of Yoga

Once you memorize the basic movements in golf, you are free to pay attention to more advanced details. You can focus on the next level of your game. The same is true with yoga. Let's now look at the structure of yoga to form a solid foundation from which to start the practice.

Yoga was originally a practice to calm the fluctuations of the mind. If each of your thousands of thoughts each day were like a wave on the ocean, you'd be navigating a stormy sea of information to sort out that which matters most to you and to make appropriate decisions. The ride could be rough and exhausting.

The 8 Limbs of Yoga

1. Ethical behaviors for thriving relationships *Yamas*

Extend kindness. Speak truthfully. Be generous. Conserve your energy. Skip jealousy. You earn the trust of fellow players when you live the yamas on the golf course. You likely do this already by complimenting an excellent shot or modifying your stroke count on the previous hole (Darn, you forgot that miss with your approach wedge and scored a 6 instead of a 5). You also give honors to the player with the best score on the previous hole.

2. Inner habits that build character *Niyamas*

Keep clean (body and mind). Study yourself. Be content. Cultivate discipline. Surrender. Niyamas elevate your self-respect and happiness. They foster a sense of control that inspires others. Perhaps you remain tranquil when hit up on by the group behind you and stay the most confident golfer in your foursome during an unexpected rain shower. When you embody the niyamas, you can simultaneously accept yourself where you're at while making strides for improvement (and have a lot more fun on the journey, too).

3. Physical yoga postures *Asana*

Each specific movement on the yoga mat increases the health of the spine. You fold forward, bend laterally, extend, twist, and invert. From these five categories, thousands of postures are possible in a given yoga class. The trick is to know how to sequence them to reach your goals. Later in this book, I'll help you get started with postures that get you focused before a round and recover after one.

4. Deliberate breathing techniques *Pranayama*

Just like yoga poses, certain breathing patterns can be used to produce a specific result. Need to wake up for your game? Lengthen the inhale. Calm your nerves? Change your exhale. I'll cover how to do this—and much more—to maximize your energy on the course.

5. Tune out distractions *Pratyahara*
This is how you avoid shanking the ball right 90-degrees into the marshal's cart when he pulls up alongside your group or how you prevent missing the ball entirely. You might be way past those errors, but the techniques of focus you learn in this aspect of yoga keep you playing your game no matter what goes on around you.

6. Find a focal point *Dharana*
There's a common saying that *"where your attention goes your energy flows."* This begins with the point of your gaze when your eyes are open and the intention in your mind when they're not. As you find a focal point, you have better balance on the yoga mat. You can also increase the likelihood of hitting your target on the golf course.

7. Sustained focus over time *Dhyana*
If Dharana teaches you to focus on one swing at a time, Dhyana gives you the superpower to stay present shot-by-shot the entire round. Consider it the mental match to physical endurance, avnd you build it via the practice of every other aspect of yoga.

8. Oneness, bliss, the zone *Samadhi*
Samadhi is a state where the thought and thinker dissolve into one. It's where action and awareness merge to generate an experience far beyond our normal selves. The Greeks called this *"Ecstasis."* [5] Athletes call it the flow state.[6] It is experienced on the course as a string of effortless holes. The great news is that while you can't always predict the moment you'll land in the zone, you can prepare yourself mentally and physically to be there more often. Yoga shows you how.

In yoga, you step back from the tumultuous onslaught of thoughts. Rather than being caught up in them, you simply witness them. It's like ditching your listing boat in favor of a helicopter rescue. You get to hover above the mental chatter and the ride becomes smoother. You become calmer, too.

Yoga allows you to detach your identity from *being* your thoughts and emotions to *witnessing* them as only one aspect of your broader whole.

This is another way to describe getting into the flow state.

Patanjali didn't need brain scans to know this was possible. Known as the father of modern yoga, Patanjali outlined eight steps to steady your mind.[7,8] He described this using the limbs of a tree. Since I'm a water lover, I use the analogy of a ship's wheel on the previous page to describe them instead.

Once you know your destination (or your goals), you can grab the handles anywhere you'd like and steer your body, life, and golf game in that direction with more certainty.

> "The small actions you take each day to keep learning and practice act like compound interest. If you get one percent better each day, you will end up 37% better by the end of the year!"
>
> –James Clear[9]

Tips to Start Your Practice

Samadhi is the ultimate aim of yoga. Playing in the zone is a goal on the golf course. Yet this state is unlike a college degree, where once achieved, it's yours forevermore. Achieving flow requires practice, practice, and more practice.

If you just groaned audibly, I understand.

We often view practice as tedious. After only a few repetitions, the novelty fades and you experience a thrill equivalent to that of watching paint dry. Boring! Just spend a few consecutive days on the range, and you'll be eager to play a full round.

So how is a yoga practice going to be any different?

In the big picture, it's not.

Buzzkill, I know.

But I'm a realistic optimist. Or an optimistic realist.

I know that you still have to get dressed, show up, and give it your best effort to improve at anything in life. The trick is to find the delicate balance between progress and challenge to stay motivated. We'll cover practical ways to do this in the upcoming weeks together. In the meantime, I suggest the following tips to build a strong yoga foundation from the get-go.

Tip 1: Get the Right Gear

Just like the right clubs, tees, and shoes can make your time on the course more enjoyable, there are yoga props that can enhance the time on your mat, too. I suggest you invest in the following:

- Yoga mat. There are lots of styles and sizes on the market today. Just make sure you get one that is durable and keeps you from slipping even when you're sweaty. Manduka[10] mats are known for this (and they're the brand I use).
- Pair of yoga blocks. While one is helpful, two can provide more symmetrical support during challenging poses. They amplify your sense of sturdiness, and this is true whether you purchase foam, wood, or cork blocks.
- Strap. A strap gives you additional access to yoga poses if you have limited flexibility. If you have a belt or scarf at home, that can work, too.
- Blanket(s) or towel(s) provide extra padding for sensitive knee joints, and they can elevate the hips when in seated postures. Plus, they can add more comfort to poses used in the recovery portion of this program.

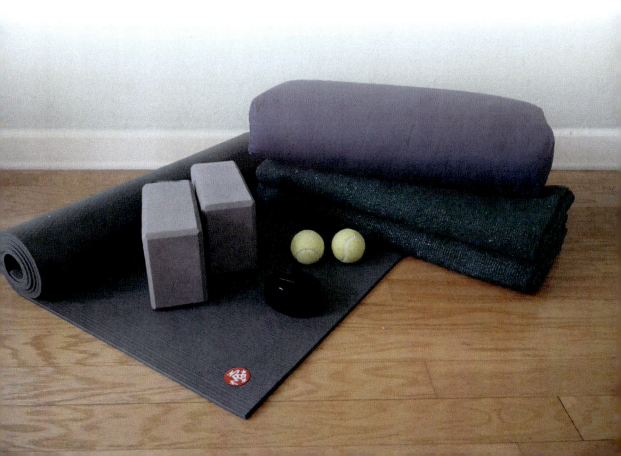

- Folding chair. Yoga is for *every* body, even if you can't take yoga poses on the floor. That's when chair yoga is an alternate way to practice. Check out the sequence on page 163 for ideas on how to use a chair in yoga.
- Two tennis balls. While you might not play this sport, tennis balls are a handy piece of equipment to have around your house for yoga. Mainly, they help remove stored tension. We'll explore this in week 5.

Tip 2: Carve Out Space to Practice

Once you have the gear, you'll need to carve out space to practice. By this, I mean time on your calendar and a place to unroll your yoga mat. If you don't, your gear will likely end up as a dusty collection piece stored in the garage next to that set of skis you swore you were going to use this year (only you forgot to … again).

I suggest you pull out your planner now and see what you've got scheduled for the next two months. Notice what days you regularly play golf. Look for gaps between activities and see where you could possibly squeeze in the lessons from this book. I suggest you reserve 30- or 60-minute blocks of time to get on the yoga mat. Or, you can wait and do your planning on a week-by-week basis.

Just remember that you're far more likely to show up for an event, even a yoga date with yourself, if you have it scheduled on your calendar in advance.

As for the best place to practice yoga?

Any room in your house that has hard-surface flooring works best. It could be tile, hardwood, or even firm carpet. And since you'll be moving in yoga, I recommend you remove any objects within a six- or eight-foot radius of your mat. That way you're less likely to get hurt should you lose your balance during class.

Tip 3: Show Up

One of my favorite quotes is *"the cost of a book includes the price tag plus the time required to read it."* A yoga mat is the same. You now have the gear and time reserved on the calendar. It's time to cash in on your investment and begin your practice. Simply unroll your mat. Commit to doing your best, free yourself of preconceived expectations, and have fun learning something new.

Tip 4: Listen to Your Body

Many exercise programs encourage you to push through pain to get results. I know many athletes who live with this mindset. I did myself for years. I pushed past warning signs of fatigue and ended up breaking a collarbone with a layout catch in the endzone during an Ultimate Frisbee match. This compromised my ability to do anything with my shoulder, from brushing my hair to playing volleyball, for far too long.

Thankfully, yoga changed my approach to training.

Yoga encourages you to listen to your body and understand the subtle signals being sent to your brain in any given movement. You'll get feedback to ease up or to breathe deeper, to slow down or speed up.

You just need to pay attention.

The most important thing is that you stay out of pain!

You might experience dull, pulling sensations that indicate you're moving your body in unfamiliar ways. But *never* should you feel a sharp, burning, or piercing sensation. This is your cue to exit a pose immediately.

Once you're out of pain you can assess why it arose in the first place. You can revisit the same pose with the use of props or assume an alternate pose. I'll provide lots of options throughout this book to help you target the same golf-related areas of the body. The goal is to use the pose that keeps you free of pain.

Tip 5: Be Patient as You Learn the Basics

In my first golf lesson, I was eager to hit the range and learn the full-swing. Only we walked over to the putting green instead. I was disappointed and worried that golf would be just another boring activity, like that snooze-fest of a yoga class I took years ago.

Given that we use a putter roughly 40% of the time during a round, I have come to respect the importance of this stroke.

I just needed to have more patience when learning the basics of golf, and I propose you do the same on the yoga mat. As you gain confidence and mastery of those fundamentals, you can then increase the challenge accordingly.

> *"It is only when correct practice is followed for a long time, without interruptions and with a positive attitude of eagerness, that you can succeed."*
>
> –Patanjali, Indian sage and author

Tip 6: Find Your Edge

Finding your edge is how you decipher the degree of challenge that is appropriate for you. It's like the Goldilocks principle. If you try too little or don't experience enough resistance, you'll lose interest. Your skills won't improve either. Or if a yoga practice becomes too difficult, you'll likely get discouraged, frustrated, or worse, injured.

Your goal is to find that sweet spot of challenge. You want to be able to breathe deeply, while simultaneously aware of new sensations in the body. Said another way, your breath will help you find your limit on the yoga mat—and indicate when you've pushed beyond it.

Tip 7: Enjoy the Process

This last tip might be the most obvious of them all. You want practice to be fun. You want the process to be as satisfying and pleasurable as possible so you stay motivated long-term.

Just think about how you do this on the golf course. You chat with friends or buy a round of drinks to make the day more enjoyable. Or during practice, you transform mundane drills into games on the range to be more playful.

To make a yoga practice more fun, I smile a lot. I laugh when encountering a challenge. At home, I place my yoga mat near the window so I can watch squirrels chasing each other around the large oak tree in the yard. This reminds me not to take myself, or any yoga pose, too seriously.

If you spend any time around a small child, you'll notice they naturally include a sense of whimsy in their actions. We can do the same as adults on the mat, too. Simply observe which elements of yoga you enjoy, which styles leave you feeling the best, and repeat those frequently to build a sustainable practice.

Activity: The Flexible Golfer Questionnaire

Answer the questions below to determine how this book can elevate your golf game, health, and overall quality of life. I suggest you use a blank sheet of paper or a journal for this activity. You can then update your responses as you progress over the upcoming weeks, and at the end of this program.

Primary Aim

1. What do you value most in life?

2. How does golf fit into that picture?

3. How does your health fit into your larger life aim?

4. What kind of person do you want to be (on and off the course)?

Golf Goals

5. What are the best technical aspects of your game? Which need improvement?

6. What would you like to achieve in the next 6 months with your golf game?

7. What steps are you ready and willing to take to make that happen?

Yoga Goals

8. How often do you step out of your comfort zone to grow?

9. What physical transformation would you like yoga to help you achieve (on and off the course)?

10. In what ways would you like to improve your focus in your life and golf game?

11. Which friend(s) can you share this information with in the coming weeks and months to increase your accountability and joy in the learning process?

Putting it Together

Yoga is a pathway to increase physical health, focus the mind, and explore your potential. It's a practice that enhances your flexibility, but doesn't require you to be flexible before you begin. Yoga is also a fantastic training tool to improve your golf game. This is because yoga:

- Increases mobility (you gain flexibility with control)
- Boosts your balance (for a steadier golf swing)
- Enhances body awareness (which can prevent injury)
- Builds strength and power (to get more yardage with each shot)
- Heightens your focus (for more clarity and confidence on the course)

Take Action Now

- ❑ **Order your yoga equipment.**
  Revisit the gear you'll need to start a yoga practice and purchase those items now.

- ❑ **Schedule time to learn.**
  Pull out your calendar to check two things: one, that you've got time available to read this book each week, and two, the time to get on the yoga mat and internalize your learning moving forward. The suggested amount of practice time is outlined in the corresponding lessons.

- ❑ **Start with clarity.**
  Complete the questionnaire on the previous pages to highlight any outcomes you want to achieve by reading this book (and how to track your priorities along the way).

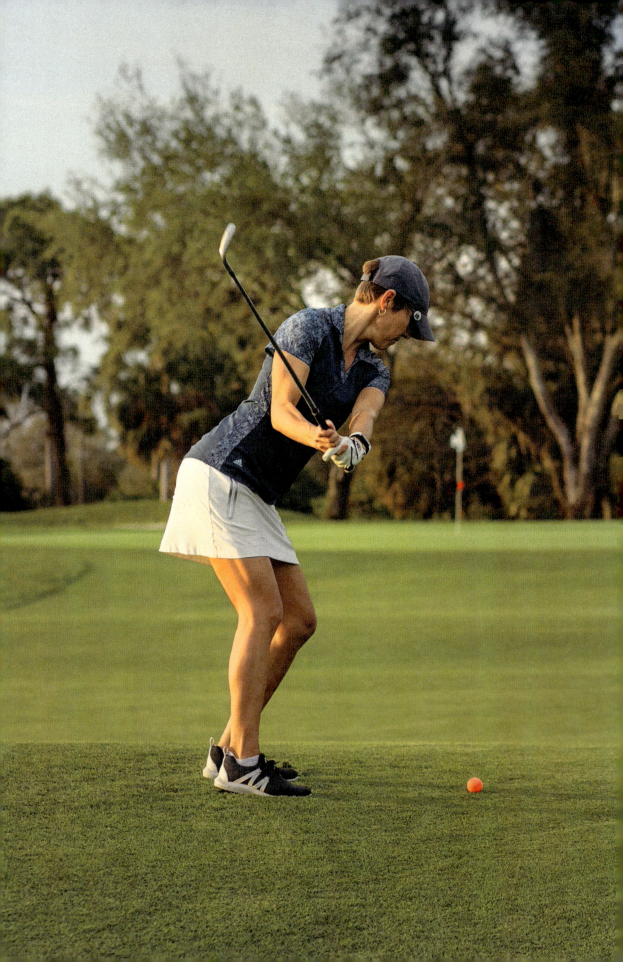

WEEK 1

Discover the Golf-Body in Motion

"The golf swing requires more than 300 joints in the body to move through significant portions of their range of motion, and each one of the body's 640 [skeletal] muscles to perform at a high level."

—Dr. Craig Davies

WEEK 1 OVERVIEW

Human anatomy is a complex subject. Yet, we simplify it this week, so you know what's going on internally as you swing your club. This allows you to create the most efficient swing possible, thwart injuries, and incorporate yoga in a way that's right for you.

The objective of golf is deceivingly simple: play all 18 holes with as few strokes as possible. And success hinges largely on one foundational element: your swing. I knew this from the moment I picked up a golf club to simply test my interest in the sport, which is why I hired a coach from the get-go.

This was for three reasons. First, the golf swing is tough. It's unnatural. Why waste time with poor mechanics and make the game more challenging than it already is? Two, I wanted to enjoy playing the game with Steve, and I knew learning the basics from him could strain our relationship. And three, I wanted to be good from the start.

This made me the ideal client. I was eager to absorb information about hand positions, swing planes, and rhythm. I had no previous experience to revise or undo. In other words, I was fresh, moldable clay.

Come to find out, not everyone approaches learning this way. My friend, Marilyn, was already playing when she sought out the same coach. She didn't want to change her putting stroke to make it more mechanical. She liked the feel of her grip and stance. Why change what was already working?

Whether you fall into the *"perfect-swing-mechanics"* camp or the *"I-love-my-personal-swing"* group[1], the asymmetrical movement to swing a club is taxing on your body.

It involves many moving parts crossing various planes in space. You must get your bones and joints to move in a coordinated manner to generate power. You need your muscles working at a high capacity and to operate with precision. Said in a simpler way: A coordinated and powerful golf swing results from an integrated chain of accurate movements.[2]

This involves training your muscles to activate when needed and rest when they're not to increase the efficiency of your swing. When I say efficient, I mean we're going to improve the communication between various parts of your body so they can work systematically to produce a strong, consistent swing—one that is repeatable and less prone to injury. I'll teach you how to do this in a safe and progressive way throughout this book.

If you're more efficient with your swing, you also save energy. Imagine what you could do with that extra energy in your golf game. You'd have more brainpower to select the best club for your next shot or decipher the perfect line to sink your putt. More strength and stamina could mean extra yardage with your drives. This energetic reserve might also be the ingredient that transforms an average round into a great one!

Start with the Feet

A coordinated swing starts with your feet. The feet are full of sensory receptors that collect data from the ground beneath you and then relay that information to the brain. Corresponding muscles, tendons, and ligaments activate as a result to keep you balanced.

This all occurs in milliseconds and is done without you having to consciously think about it.

Yet, you can deliberately pay attention to your feet before taking your swing to establish a solid foundation. You can focus on a grounded, stable stance. Then, you can press your feet into the earth. This initiates ground reactive force which, thanks to the laws of physics, results in the ground pushing back with an equal amount of force.

This force is then transferred up the body. It moves through the legs, pelvis, and spine, then out to your club and, ultimately, the golf ball. When you relay this transmission of energy in an orderly way, you get more power and distance with each shot. This means that the actions of your feet affect the entire chain of kinetic energy in your body and the quality of your golf shot as a whole.

Yoga teaches you to increase awareness at the feet. You can start this now by observing the sensations around your feet. What textures are in contact with the soles of your feet? Are your feet currently in socks or shoes? What is the temperature of the surface beneath your feet?

To heighten this awareness even more—and to prepare them for the golf swing—use the exercise on the following page.

Activity: Activate the Feet

To activate the feet, you'll move from a flat-footed, neutral position to one in which the feet are flexed. The arm options in this activity are optional. They simply offer more of a challenge. I recommend trying this activity with bare feet first. Then you can then repeat these movements in golf shoes before your next round.

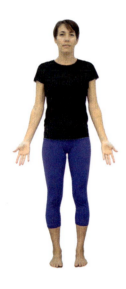

Start in Mountain Pose

- Stand with your feet hip-distance apart, with the feet parallel and all 10 toes pointing forward.[3]
- Press your feet down into the floor. Press through the ball mount of each foot, and the heel as well. See if you can imagine equal pressure pushing down from the right and left sides of each foot. Remain light on the toes.
- Lift the quadriceps away from the kneecaps. Notice how the legs start to activate.
- Keep the hips level in space, and imagine the spine growing taller as the crown of the head lightly lifts toward the ceiling.
- Broaden the collarbones and relax the shoulders, moving the shoulder blades down and away from your ears.

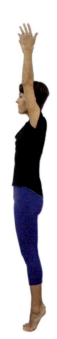

Shift Your Weight

- Begin to rock your body weight to the front half of each foot without lifting the heels away from the floor.
- Then, rock your weight back without lifting your toes.
- Rock back and forth a few times to create more sensation throughout your feet. Return to a balanced position before moving on.

Lift the Heels and Arms Simultaneously

- As you inhale, shift weight toward the ball of each foot and lift the heels away from the floor. Distribute your weight evenly between the inside and outside edges of the foot and prevent excess downward pressure on the toes. A whole host of muscles in the feet and legs make this motion possible.

- At the same time, raise your arms in front of you. This movement activates the chest and shoulder muscles.
- As you finish the inhale, come to your highest point of balance. Your arms can end parallel to the floor or up by your ears.

Lower Heels and Arms on the Exhale
- As you breathe out, return your arms to your side and the heels to the ground at the same time. This movement increases cellular communication between muscle groups, too.

Repeat this exercise 10-15 times to activate the feet. Then stand in Mountain Pose for a few cycles of breath when done. Become aware of any new sensations in the body.

To make this activity more challenging...
- Keep your heels and arms lifted to any degree you find comfortable. Lower the hips toward the ground in a balancing Chair Pose.
- Hold this position for 3-5 cycles of breath. Then, either keep the heels lifted as you raise the hips or drop them to the ground as you return to a flat-footed Mountain Pose.
- You can repeat this balancing chair pose 5-10 times to warm up the feet and legs.

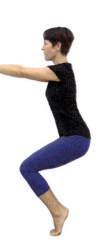

Ready Position

Ready position is the grounded stance from which you set your club in motion. The feet get activated first. Then the rest of your body turns on to ensure a steady swing. Here's how:

Flex the ankles. In this position, the top of your feet moves closer to the shins, and the front of the lower legs engage. The calf muscles on the lower back portion of your legs elongate at the same time. This changes if you stand on the side of a hill with a downhill lie. Yet, in general, your ankles will be in this flexed ready position.

Bend your knees. Your knee joint is a complex structure of bone, cartilage, ligaments, and tendons connecting to muscles. Knee flexion—or bending your knees—activates several muscles on the back of your thigh as well as some supporting muscles in your inner front thigh. We'll strengthen these with various yoga postures.

Flex the hips. Your hips are the junction where the lower and upper body meet, and they are slightly flexed in a ready position. You tilt the pelvis moderately forward to hinge the torso over the ball, requiring core strength, muscular engagement at the front of the hips and thighs, and a lengthening at the back of the legs.

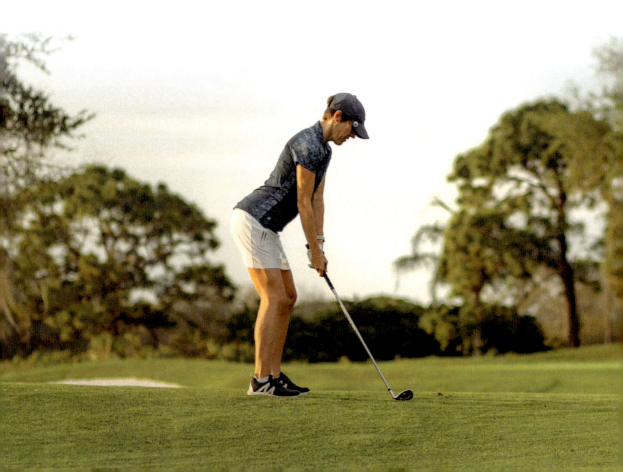

Keep the spine neutral. This means the natural curve found at each portion of your spine stays intact.

Protract the shoulder blades. Your shoulder blades move slightly apart and forward, so you can grip your club and keep it in place. You will memorize this sensation using the activity on page 42.

Flex the shoulders. Think about this for a moment. When you stand up straight, with your arms by your side, the arms are in a neutral position. If you remain upright, and start to lift your arms forward, the shoulders flex. Now hinge at the torso, and you're ready to hold your club and hit the ball. The small muscles of your deltoid make this initial shoulder flexion possible.

Engage the arms and hands, which allows you to grip your club.

Keep the head and neck neutral. The muscles that support the head and neck will be working a bit harder in a ready position since your spine is more forward in space (and you're fighting gravity). Yoga helps build more strength in this region. Yoga is also a great tool to release unwanted tension that often accumulates in the neck from playing golf.

Engage the entire back of the body— from heel to head—to prevent falling forward in this ready position. You'll utilize these same muscles again as you begin your takeaway.

The Backswing

Now it's time to coordinate these segments of your body into an efficient backswing. This requires flexibility in your muscles to create a greater range of motion with your joints. You also want to have control as you move. That's called mobility, remember?

With greater mobility, you harness more potential energy up the spine—a power that can then be unleashed from the top of your backswing into a forceful downswing. Let's take a look at how your body comes to life as you pull the club away from the ball.

The Feet

As you initiate your upswing, your weight will transfer slightly to the inside of your back foot while keeping the front foot equally grounded. Activating, or contracting, your quadriceps also helps the downward pressure of the feet.

The Hips

The hip joint is responsible for our ability to walk, run, and jump. Strength in this region is important during the backswing for two main reasons. First, the hips bear the brunt of your body weight. Secondly, strong hips allow you to remain steady as you pull the club away. This prevents a lateral sway in the hips that could lead to inconsistent and errant shots.

The muscles you want to be strong and stable around the hip joint during your takeaway include the:
- Quadriceps (quads) and hip flexors
- Hamstrings
- Gluteus medius and maximus
- Deep muscles of the core

It's from this strength that you then turn the pelvis away from the golf ball. Your trail leg, or back leg, internally rotates to make this possible. The problem is that your hips will sway side-to-side if you don't have enough hip flexibility to do this.

We'll use yoga poses to amplify strength and flexibility in your hips to generate a more reliable backswing in your game. For now, let's start by stabilizing the hips with the yoga movements up next.

> *"The majority of the benefits that come from a yoga practice come from very simple things like paying attention, taking a deep breath, or listening to the body. They don't come from really hard poses. Hard poses are fun and interesting and valuable, too. Yet a majority of the benefits of a yoga practice come from the simple things."*
>
> –Jason Crandell, yoga teacher

Activity: Stabilize the Hips

This toe-tapping activity builds strength in the outer hip muscles and improves your overall balance.

Begin in Chair Pose

- From Mountain Pose, sink the hips down like you would sit in a chair. Tuck the tailbone slightly and elongate the low back. Move the knees back in space so you can glance down at your toes (which should be pointing forward). As you bring more weight into the heels, counter that with downward pressure in the front half of each foot to keep you balanced.
- Draw the belly button toward the spine to engage the core.
- Keep your chest facing forward as much as possible.
- Place your hands on your hips for added support. This also prevents the pelvis from tilting side-to-side as you move.

Tap Your Toes to the Side

- Bring more weight onto your left foot and unweight your right foot.
- Sustain a level pelvis as you lift the right foot entirely off the ground and tap the toes on your right foot out to the side. Go only as far as you can while keeping your left knee pointed forward and your hips steady.
- Then tap the toes back to where the right foot was initially. Only this time, don't set the foot down.
- Repeat 10-15 sets of toe-taps on the right foot, then repeat on the left side.

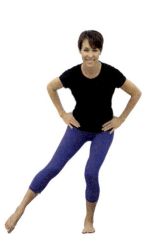

Rest in Mountain Pose when you are done. Observe any changes in the legs.

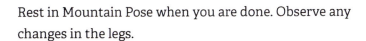

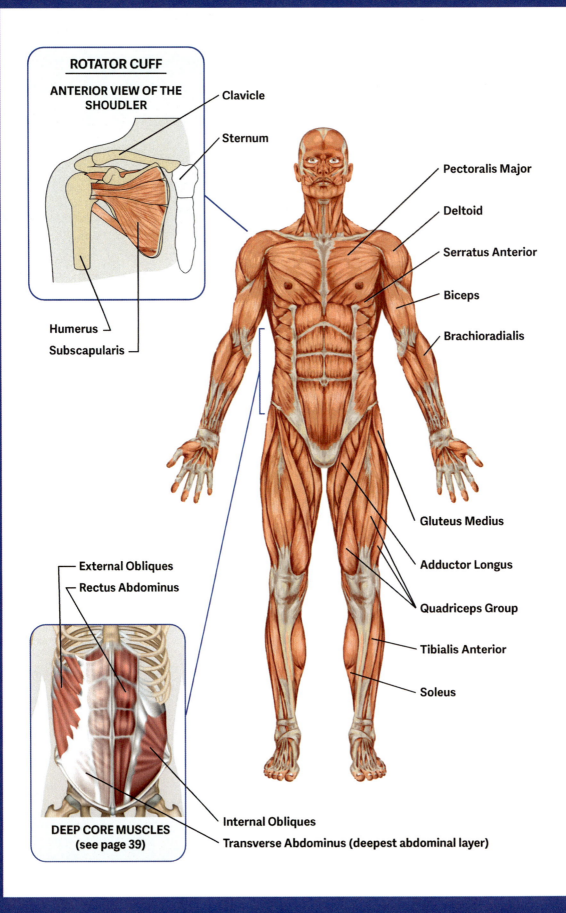

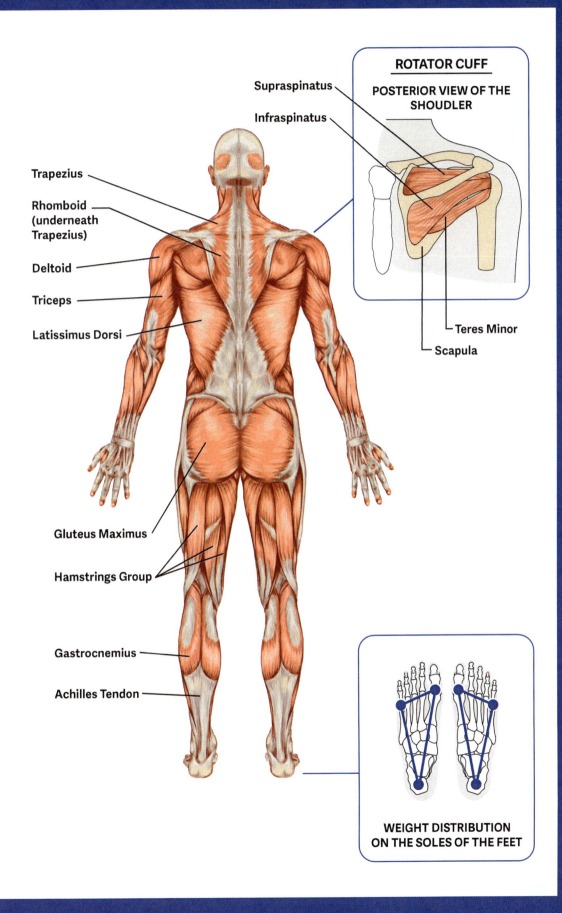

The Spine

Good posture, also known as proper alignment of the spine, is essential for you to move in optimal ways. If you look at the diagram below, your spine has natural curves that form an S-shape when viewed from the side. The spine's cervical and lumbar regions have a lordotic or a slight inward curve, and the thoracic spine and sacrum have a kyphotic or gentle outward curve. These curves work together like a coiled spring to absorb shock as you move. And when in proper alignment, unwanted wear and tear on supportive structures around the spine is reduced.

Good posture sets you up for a consistent and powerful golf swing, too.

Your core muscles engage as you hinge forward to stand over your ball in a ready position. Then you keep your natural spinal curves intact as you rotate into your backswing. This way, you gather a tremendous amount of energy to unleash into your downswing. You also generate more ball speed upon contact.

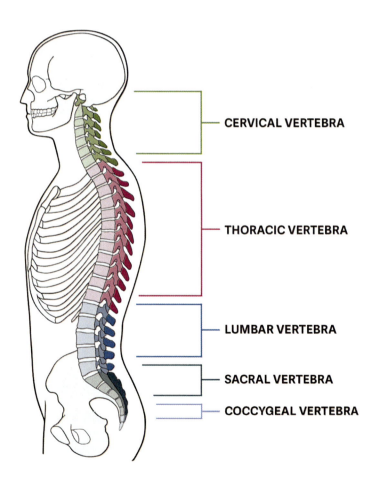

In simple terms, proper spinal alignment in your backswing amplifies your accuracy and power during each shot, all while minimizing your risk of injury.

So which muscles help you do this?

The short, thick, and deep muscles along the lumbar spine allow you to twist, as do larger muscles of your abdominals and latissimus dorsi (lats). What's amazing is that the muscles on the target side of your body must be long and strong to make rotation possible.

Yoga is one of the best ways to build strength in each of these groups and offset the low back pain that plagues many golfers. We'll also use various postures to elongate these tissues to get you into a more efficient backswing position.

Quick Review of the Core

Here are the four basic muscle groups that comprise the abdominals. You can also view them on page 36.

1. **Transversus abdominis**, the deepest layer, runs horizontally across the abdomen and wraps around the entire torso from front to back. It also connects the ribs and pelvis. This corset-like muscle group maintains internal abdominal pressure, stabilizes your entire midsection, and is recruited almost any time a limb of the body moves.

2. The **rectus abdominis** is a long, flat muscle positioned between the ribs and pubic bone at the front of the pelvis. It is responsible for flexing the lumbar spine, tilting the pelvis, and aiding in respiration.

3. **External obliques** are located on each side of the rectus abdominis, moving from the ribs down to the iliac crest of the pelvis. They allow body-twisting movements to the opposite side.

4. **Internal obliques** run upwards from the hip bones to the midline of the body. They work in conjunction with the diaphragm for respiration, help your body bend laterally, and perform same-side twisting motions.

Activity: Engage the Core

A strong core, which includes all the musculature around the midsection, protects the spine during a powerful golf swing. This version of foot-tapping builds muscle memory here in a functional way.

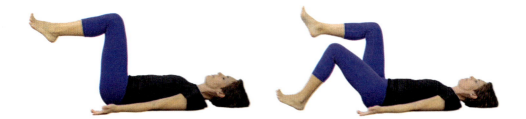

Start on Your Back
- Notice the back of your pelvis heavy and your belly button dropping down toward the spine. This initiates a subtle abdominal contraction from the get-go.
- Draw your knees toward your chest. Stop once they stack directly over the hips. The shins will then move parallel to the floor, resulting in a 90-degree angle at the knee joint.
- The core will engage to a higher degree to keep you in this position.
- Sustain a neutral spine as you relax the muscles of the face, neck, shoulders, and anywhere else in the body that doesn't need to help keep your legs steady.
- Stay and breathe here for 30-60 seconds if you are challenged enough.

Tap Your Toes Toward the Floor
- To intensify this activity, keep your knees bent 90-degrees. The left leg stays as is. On an inhale, move your right knee forward and lower the right heel toward the floor. It might even tap the floor lightly.
- Only go as far as you can while keeping the natural curves of your spine intact and your breathing steady.
- Exhale and draw the right knee back to your starting position.
- Repeat on the left side.

Complete 5-10 rounds on each side, and hug both knees in toward the chest when you're done.

The Shoulders

From stable hips, your spine can rotate away from the ball, and your shoulders can mobilize to reach the top of your backswing. Given that your shoulders have the widest range of motion in the entire body, they are also the most prone to injury. That's why you want flexibility and control in the surrounding muscles of this joint.

Yoga will give you this mobility. Yet, in order to understand how the various postures will do this, let's take a quick look into the anatomy of your shoulders.

Three bones comprise each shoulder girdle.

- The scapula (or shoulder blades)
- The clavicle (or collar bones)
- The humerus (or upper arm bones)

The rotator cuff muscles—the subscapularis, infraspinatus, teres minor, and supraspinatus (SITS)—are the deepest and provide stability for the shoulder. They also help you move in small, refined ways.

Then you have larger muscles around the shoulder complex that are responsible for larger movements like your backswing. These muscles include the deltoids, rhomboids, lats, trapezius (traps), serratus anterior, and pectoralis major (pecs).

You don't have to memorize the fancy scientific names for these muscles. I share them so you can recognize (and appreciate) that many moving parts in the upper body require tone and stamina to complete the golf swing. Also, you'll then have a point of reference when we train these areas on the yoga mat.

The most obvious of these muscles are your deltoids. These engage as you flex the shoulders to lift your club away from your body and away from the ground.

What often gets overlooked, though, is the movement necessary around your shoulder blades to hold your club at the top of your backswing. The lead shoulder blade, the one closest to the target, moves forward in space so that the front arm can pull back in the upswing. The trail shoulder blade, which is the one furthest from the target, retracts and moves closer to the spine, allowing the back arm to get into the proper position.

We'll start by using the upcoming activity to mobilize the shoulder blades in this way.

Activity: Mobilize the Shoulder Blades

Even though the shoulder blades can move in many directions, this activity focuses on two specific actions: protraction, or pushing the shoulder blades forward, and retraction, drawing them closer to the spine. This gives you greater control and prevents injuries in your golf swing.

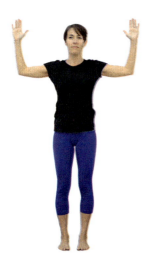

Make Cactus Arms

- Start in Mountain Pose.
- Make a cactus shape with your arms. The upper arms will be parallel to the ground, and the lower arms will be vertical. Have your palms facing forward.
- Keep your spine neutral and your front ribs drawn in. Without changing the shape of your arms, move your Cactus Arms back in space. This movement will force the shoulder blades closer to the spine (retraction). You might even notice the skin between your shoulder blades and spine begin to wrinkle. That's a good thing!

Follow with Eagle Arms

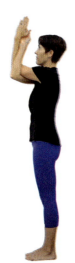

- As you exhale, it's time to move the Cactus Arms forward. Bring the elbows and forearms as close together as possible while maintaining a 90-degree angle at the elbow. Your shoulder blades will move apart as a result (protraction). Then simultaneously drop the shoulders down and away from the ears, lift the elbows away from the floor, and push the elbows slightly away from the body. The upper arm bones will stay parallel to the floor as you do this.
- Stay in this position if you already notice a stretch between the shoulder blades. To intensify the stretch, place one elbow on top of the other.
- For a further challenge, draw the back of the forearms toward one another and bring the palms to touch.

The Downswing

Just like the backswing, your downswing involves a methodical chain of movements in the body. Only instead of coiling energy upward, you're going to uncoil it downward. This energy is at its peak at the top of your backswing, and its potential can only be fully realized when the downswing is done properly.

This starts with the feet. The lead foot presses down into the ground, which initiates the ground reactive force and begins to transfer the weight to the target side of your body. If you're a right-handed golfer, your left foot presses down and positions the left knee over the left foot. If you're a leftie, you transfer weight to your right foot and position your right knee over your right foot.

Then the very same hip stabilizing muscles you used to steady the pelvis in the backswing will generate force in the downswing. Your glutes and external hip rotators initiate the turn of the hips toward your target. The quadriceps help straighten the knee to push the ground away. And the hamstrings and glutes extend the hips and pelvis forward. The trail leg, which is the back leg, utilizes many muscles to help drive your weight to the front foot. Your quadriceps, hamstrings, and glutes activate on that back leg to make this possible.

Then, as your hips clear, the arms can move into position.

You use larger muscles around the shoulder, such as the lats, to amplify power to your downswing. The lats, which attach to the pelvis, spine, and upper arm bone, are phenomenal pulling muscles. They're also used in other sports such as rowing or cross-country skiing to propel the body forward. On the golf course, the lats on your lead side pull your body and club toward your target.

The pecs, which reside on the front side of your body, counter the force of the downswing to help stabilize your shoulder complex while it's in motion. Even the forearms, wrists, and hand muscles must engage to provide you with a solid grip in the downswing. This is especially important when you're hitting out of long or thick grass.

The yoga poses in this program establish muscle memory in these muscles independently. Better still, you'll train them to activate in conjunction with one another so that you have a more efficient and coordinated downswing. This translates to more precision, power, and distance with each shot.

The Follow-Through

Now that you've generated a significant amount of speed and force in the downswing, it's time to bring your body to a halt. That's where the follow-through enters the picture. Many golfers overlook the importance of the follow-through because it's not as flashy as the downswing. They also underestimate how taxing the follow-through is on the body.

Many of your joints are at the end range of their capacity and the muscular tissue that supports these joints must work at a higher percentage of their maximum output to slow you down. Put another way, these muscles need to be long and strong at the same time to help you decelerate. This includes your:

- Serratus anterior, rhomboids, lats, pecs, and rotator cuff muscles to stabilize the shoulders
- Core muscle to protect the spine
- Hip stabilizers to keep you steady

And don't forget your feet!

As you pivot into the finishing phase of your follow-through, your big toe extends in order to get the rest of your foot and hips into the proper position. If your big toe can't extend properly for some reason, whether that be for neurological reasons or simply due to limited range of motion, the low back will engage to complete the golf swing. This can lead to unwanted injuries.

That's why we'll use yoga to boost flexibility in the toes, just as we do in the rest of the body. We'll also build strength throughout your musculature so you can complete all phases of your golf swing safely.

Problems That Hinder a Golf Swing

In addition to limited flexibility or decreased strength, there are other factors that could hinder the efficiency of your swing. These include:

Limited Movement

The first is that the golf swing requires you to move through all three planes of motion, only you don't move throughout each of them on a regular basis. Because of the position of our eyes, we move forward and backward more frequently. You twist or bend laterally far less often in everyday life. Thankfully, you'll move through all three planes deliberately on your yoga mat to prepare you for the golf swing.

Age-Related Issues

Another reason your swing is less-than-optimal could be due to the general stiffness that comes with age. Synovial fluid, the natural lubricant that allows your joints to move, decreases over time. Your cartilage tends to thin, too. Physical activity, like a yoga practice, can offset many of these changes and keep you more mobile on the course.

Poor Posture

Our modern lifestyle also lends to poor posture. Many of my waking hours are spent in a seated position at work (even though I vary my position from a kneeling chair to a stool). You might also log numerous hours driving, reading, or watching television. And unless you live under a rock, you use your cell phone. A lot! This use of technology can place undue strain on your upper spine and compromise your posture over time.

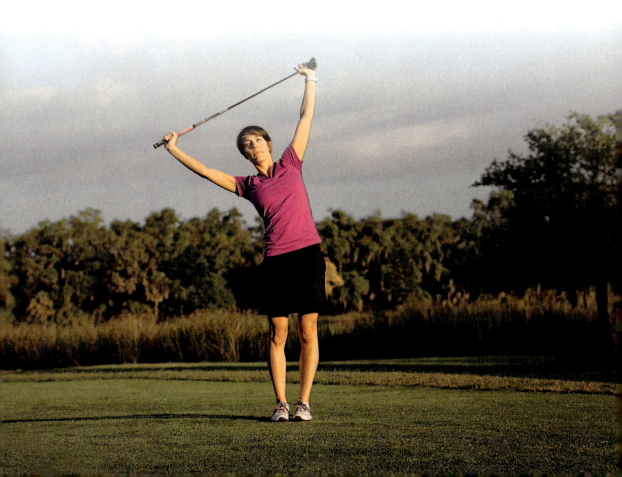

You also have gravity to deal with, which pulls everything toward the center of the Earth. These elements—combined with the above physical limitations—can all increase joint degeneration and limit your ability to swing the golf club well.

But don't think for a second that age or lack of exercise are the only limiting factors to your swing. There are a few others that can affect your mobility.

Injury

An injury or overworked muscle group can lead to weakness in the body. This deficiency can affect your range of motion, strength, or even body awareness. What also happens is that other body parts step in to compensate for this weakness. This causes your fascia to adapt in unhealthy ways, too, and generates a greater overall imbalance in your muscular tissue. As a short-term solution, this allows you to maintain bodily function. Over the long run, this can hinder your potential to swing well.

Hypermobility

Another limitation of an optimal golf swing is hypermobility. This heightened level of flexibility provides more freedom on the yoga mat, and it can help you get into a more vertical golf swing. However, if you lack control in your movements, you still run the risk of injury on the course. That's why we focus on building strength with yoga if you're hypermobile.

Developmental Delay

Even junior golfers in a growth spurt can have trouble with their golf swing. Rapid growth might create a temporary setback or decrease in performance until they adapt to their new physical size, shape, and strength.

Regardless of the physical limitation(s) hindering you right now, yoga can be used to increase your mobility and can change your swing for the better.

Putting it Together

Your body has immense potential for movement. You can recognize this via your daily activities and through the repetition of a powerful golf swing. Breaking down the various parts of the swing can also amplify your appreciation of how your body moves through it.

Yoga helps increase this potential. It helps prepare your body in a progressive, safe, and efficient manner for the powerful golf swing. And, it gives you the control to strike with precision and slow down safely in your follow-through.

Take Action Now

- ❑ **Build subtle strength first.**
  Set aside three segments of time this week to activate the feet, stabilize the hips, engage the core, and mobilize the shoulder blades. This will build muscle memory, and these movements only require 15-20 minutes when done in sequence.

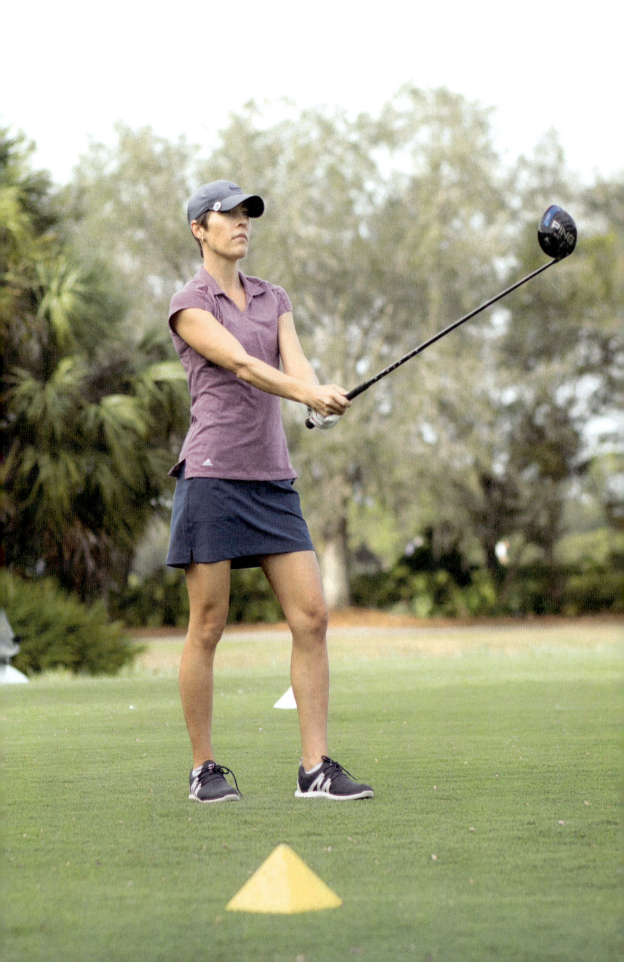

WEEK 2

Flex the Muscles of Your Mind

"No matter what a player's handicap, the scores will always be lower if the golfer thinks well."

–Tom Kite, professional golfer

WEEK 2 OVERVIEW

Improvement on the golf course is preceded by changes in the way you move and think. That's why this week, you will learn how to break negative cycles that keep you stuck in sameness and embrace the mental skills that elevate your game.

I mentioned earlier that I wasn't great at yoga when I began. Nor was I at golf. Both challenged me physically and mentally, and I knew that I'd have to adopt some basic skills if I wanted to get good at either. So, I started taking regular yoga classes under the expert eye of a seasoned instructor. I also hired a golf coach to learn the fundamentals of the game. To this day, I still work with a golf pro to refine my skills as I progress.

Ongoing improvement requires making changes. It involves transforming who you are now into the person and golfer you wish to become.

As you read these words, your brain cells are making new connections. You're already in the process of change because the brain is an organ of change. In neuroscience, this is called neuroplasticity.[1] Even the gray matter of your brain reorganizes as you alter your behavior.

Think of it this way: when you change your mind, the brain and body change, too.

I notice that very few golfers spend time learning or practicing skills that boost their focus. They don't flex the muscles of their mind. They don't build mental stamina. These very same people then get upset at themselves when they underperform on the course. This is despite the fact that they know golf is 90% mental.

I like that you're not leaving this process up to chance. You're ready to change on purpose.

So, this week, we're going to discover how to use your mind to improve your golf game. You're going to uncover what prevented you from making changes in the past, and you'll begin to consciously break old patterns. As a result, you'll have more energy and joy to embrace the new you—the you that's a better spouse, friend, parent, boss, employee, and golfer.

The Mind, Brain, and Body Connection

Humans are complex beings made up of unique thoughts, dreams, feelings, and memories. We have specific skills, interests, and habits. Each of these manifests as connections between any number of the 100 billion nerve cells in the brain. They also become evident through our beliefs and actions.

Said another way, you have a mind, brain, and body that seamlessly work together to give you life. I'm going to explain the role of each of these elements. Then we'll look at strategic ways to utilize the mind, brain, and body to elicit positive change.

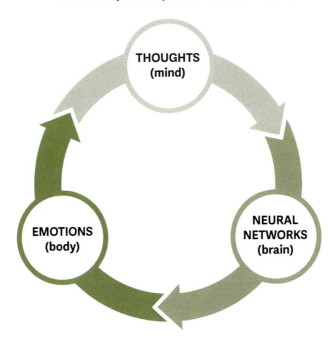

THE MIND, BRAIN, BODY CONNECTION

Mind

There are two main aspects of your mind—the conscious mind and the subconscious mind. You're probably most familiar with the conscious mind because it's how you use logic and reasoning daily.

Your conscious mind allows you to analyze your surroundings, evaluate risks, and make decisions accordingly. It's how you select a sunrise tee time over an afternoon one. It's how you choose the best playing partners. The conscious mind is also how you gauge the distance to the hole during your round and select the proper club. It even helps you refer to past memories or consider future possibilities when making these decisions.

Willpower lives in the conscious mind, too. Willpower is the vehicle through which you overcome resistance in order to take action. This is relevant to change because we're creatures of comfort. We prefer the familiar over the unknown.

Genetically, we're wired to save energy. Since starting something new requires more of your inner resources, it's easier to stay the same. Meaning, if we want to reach a new goal or improve somehow, we must get a little uncomfortable. We have to tap into faith and creativity to grow and use the intention-setting capability of the conscious mind to stay focused through it all.

Interestingly, the conscious mind doesn't fully develop until we are 7-12 years of age, and it only accounts for 5% of your total mental landscape.[2]

The real powerhouse is the subconscious mind. It processes 40 million bits of information per second and performs thousands of body functions automatically.

When we're born, we function totally from the subconscious mind. A baby soon learns that crying elicits a response from the parent to get fed or have a dirty diaper changed. This is a positive identification that becomes a behavior. Similarly, if toddlers put a hand on a hot stove, they soon link the stove—an external object—with their internal feelings of discomfort. We call those associations *"ouchie boo-boos"* in our family. In any case, a negative identification gets memorized to prevent future pain.

The subconscious mind consists of every positive and negative association made throughout your experience. These give rise to the habits, behaviors, skills, and beliefs you possess today.

While the conscious mind helps you learn something new, the subconscious stores that knowledge. This is incredibly helpful because you wouldn't want to relearn how to grip a golf club each round or how to drive a car every visit to the supermarket. In this way, the subconscious amplifies your efficiency in daily life. This only becomes problematic when your subconscious patterns run contrary to your goals. (We'll root these out with the activity on page 61.)

Brain

Each conscious or subconscious thought activates specific neural networks in the brain.[3] This nerve activity shifts the blood flow in the brain and creates measurable brain wave patterns, each of which support various body functions and correlate with different behavioral states.[4] These brain wave patterns include:

HUMAN BRAIN WAVES

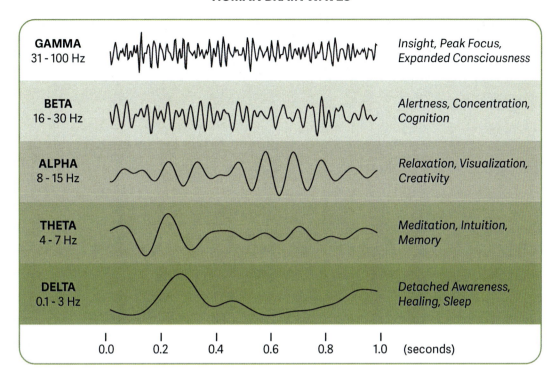

Beta: Much of your waking life is spent in the beta. Low range beta occurs when you are in a relaxed, interested state. Mid-range beta is produced when you have a sustained level of focus and some reasoning is involved. When all your senses take in stimuli from your environment and package it for greater understanding, mid-beta is present, too. High beta patterns are most evident with stress or when you're learning in a highly aroused state. These brain waves are helpful in the short-term because you can meet the unexpected demands of daily life. Yet, staying in high-beta for an extended period negatively affects your nervous system. It leads to burnout and disease.

Alpha: Your brain can slip into an alpha state from a low-range beta state when you're learning something new. Perhaps you stop to ponder a new concept in this book or daydream about your next round of golf. When this happens, you turn your attention from the outer world to the inner world. You also experience these slower brain waves when you close your eyes.

Theta: Theta waves are even slower than alpha waves. When theta patterns are present, the body is relaxed and the doorway to the subconscious opens. Maybe you've had a moment of quiet where a fresh, creative idea pops into your mind or you get inspired to take a specific action (like call an old friend). This creativity or inspiration occurred thanks to this level of brain activity.

Delta: Delta waves appear when you're in a deep sleep and the body can restore itself. There is little conscious awareness here.

Gamma: These waves are the highest frequency brain waves that occur in a highly aroused state. Only instead of being stimulated by the environment, like beta, your arousal comes from within. It's also referred to as a superconscious state.

While I don't expect you to memorize each detail of these brain wave patterns, I do want you to remember this: each type of brain wave has a direct physiological impact, and with practice, you can sense what each of these patterns feels like in the body. The yoga techniques we use throughout the book will train you how.

Body

As you think different thoughts, your brain circuits activate in corresponding sequences. A cascade of chemicals are then released into the body. If you're worried about an upcoming tournament or presentation at work, cortisol floods your system.[5] This stress hormone mobilizes your internal resources so that you can handle the perceived emergency.

If you think loving thoughts toward a family member or pet, oxytocin gets released. Theta brain waves also send serotonin throughout the body, which gives you a greater sense of inner well-being and connectedness to others.

You interpret these chemical reactions as emotions.[6] And how you feel, combined with how you think, creates your overall state of being.

The Gap

Right now, you have a current set of thoughts, beliefs, and habits about yourself as a golfer. You reinforce certain emotions each time you play. You could sustain this state of being and get more of the same. But by being here, you have committed to changing yourself, and your golf game, for the better.

To improve, you must bridge the gap between who you are right now and who you want to become.

This gap is natural. It happens throughout your life in a wide array of subjects. This desire to change for the better is how we evolve.

What I know for sure is that you would have already made the changes to your golf game if you knew what to do. Perhaps you've already worked with a pro and refined the physical skills necessary to thrive on the course.

BRIDGE THE GAP TO IMPROVE

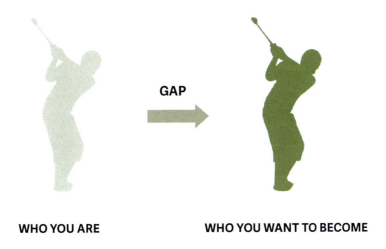

Yet, despite your hours on the range or putting green, you might still freeze up under pressure. Or you might not be making progress as quickly as you'd like. Perhaps you even sustained an injury, and you want to approach your game differently moving forward.

I'll show you why change likely eluded you in the past. Then I'll walk you through specific ways to flex the muscles of your mind, bridge the gap, and embrace positive change starting now.

What Prevents Lasting Change

According to neuroscience, your brain is organized to reflect everything you know in your environment. All your knowledge and experiences are stored in the subconscious mind and trigger the same neural pathways of the brain. This means you view your environment through the lens of past experiences.

So, let's say you're frustrated by a particular hole at your home course. It could be a particularly long hole, like #14 at my home course, Bailey Creek, which extends endlessly uphill. Or you might get frustrated with a short par 3 where you have to hit over water.

If you continuously struggle at this point in your game, you might start to repeat specific thoughts like, *"Not this hole again,"* or *"I always hit into the trees to the right,"* or *"I never play well around water."*

This thinking causes the pre-programmed neural networks in your brain to fire in incoherent patterns. Your brain waves become chaotic and uneven. They

THE NEGATIVE CYCLE OF SAMENESS

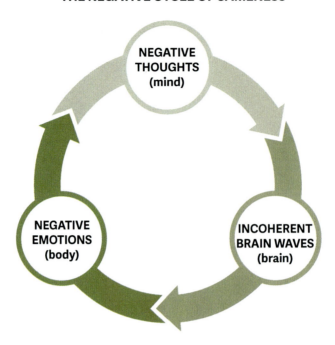

are disorderly and imbalanced. As a result of these incoherent patterns, many compartments of your brain no longer work together. This would be equivalent to each member of an orchestra playing the music they prefer instead of following the written score. The outcome is inefficient and undesirable.

Stress-related chemicals are then discharged into the body. Your adrenal glands start to pump adrenaline into your bloodstream. Your heart beats faster, your blood pressure rises, and your muscles tense up.

Each of these responses can counter your ability to relax as you stand over the ball. You likely grip your club more firmly. Or you might abandon any sense of trust in your swing altogether. This body-wide response then triggers even more doubt and frustration in the mind.

The same neural networks get activated again. Your body cells replicate to receive the same chemical messages, the same emotions. And the cycle perpetuates. It's like being stuck on a spinning hamster wheel with no escape in sight. In this pattern of sameness, it's very hard to improve.

Even if you try to use willpower to change, 5% of your conscious mind will go up against the 95% memorized patterning of the subconscious. Which do you think will win? You might get lucky every now and then or be able to keep your focus on a good thought when you're not distracted. More likely, though, you'll need to take a different approach altogether to attain lasting changes.

How to Change the Mind, Brain, or Body

You have the power to make your brain work in distinct ways because you can influence how nerve cells combine. This is done through your attention. It's your consciousness, or your conscious awareness, that recognizes unwanted patterns. It also brings the mind and body together to affect your external world (like your golf game).

According to the first law of thermodynamics, energy cannot be created or destroyed. It can only change from one form to another, which means we will take the energy you were once putting into those old habits and redirect it into new ones.

Let's break the cycle of negativity. Let's kick sameness to the curb and adventure into the new. We can start at any one of these three points—mind, brain, or body. Here's how:

Change the Mind

Thanks to the conscious mind, you can step back and objectively view your life. You can reflect on who you are and define who you want to become. As the observer, you separate yourself from your subconscious habits. You step back from the knee-jerk responses of your daily life and begin to take control once again.

Learning is one of the best ways to do this. You're already opening up to novel ideas by being here—by thinking about yourself and your golf game in unexpected ways.

No matter the medium, learning when in a relaxed state turns on the frontal lobe of your brain. This region scans your existing database of knowledge and starts to combine the stored information in new ways. It also lowers the volume

> *"It's impossible to create any new future when you are firmly rooted in your past. You have to clear away the old vestiges of the garden of the mind before you can cultivate a new self and plant seeds of new thoughts, behaviors, and emotions that create a new life."*
>
> –Dr. Joe Dispenza

of other circuits of the brain—ones that process time and space. You stay more focused in the present moment as a result.

Contemplation and introspection are additional ways you learn. Contemplation requires that you think differently about what is and imagine possibilities. With introspection, you contemplate yourself. I keep a small, blue notebook in my golf bag to jot down insights when on the course. Sometimes these are ideas directly related to my game. Many times, these thoughts are unrelated to golf. By putting pen to paper, though, I prevent these thoughts from being a distraction during my next shot.

Daydreaming is a similar mental state in which you picture the best possible outcomes. It's where you create future memories by thought alone. Ideally, you do this without the need to analyze your thoughts. We'll combine several of these elements in the activity on page 61.

Change the Brain

Every nerve cell in your brain constitutes a memory. As you step in to consciously dismantle these memories, your old self disappears. New neural networks replace old ones. Just as you would change the mind with learning, you can change the brain directly with it, too.

In a laid-back learning state, your brain waves slow down from beta to alpha. They can also move from an incoherent pattern to a coherent one. When this happens, the high and low points are parallel on an EEG. These waves are synchronized, orderly, and smooth, and all areas of the brain are highly integrated.

The goal is to memorize these states and replicate them on the golf course.

Ongoing learning is one way to do this, as mentioned above. Meditation and visualization exercises done with the eyes closed are others.

Remember, your eyes are responsible for collecting 80% of the sensory data from your environment. So, when you close them, your brain receives a signal that something is different. Your heart rate might rise at first. This is normal. Your body knows it's time to focus. It's time to pay attention.

When you close your eyes, you also remove the stimulus of people, places, and things that trigger habitual thoughts. You can't focus on the stack of bills in the office if you can't see them. Or you likely won't be distracted by a mess in the house. Without this external input, your nervous system calms down. You think less, and your brain waves slow.

Your attention shifts from outward to inward. Instead of eavesdropping on the conversation between strangers at a dinner table next to you, you hear the constant chatter of your own mind.

This doesn't mean you're crazy. We all have this inner dialogue. I became really familiar with mine when I enrolled in a 10-day silent retreat. That was like jumping into the deep end of a swimming pool before learning to swim. I would have appreciated the experience more had I known the value behind meditating in the first place. That's why I'm giving you the background here. And it's why we'll take smaller steps to change the brain throughout this book.

Change the Body

The body is perhaps the most obvious place to break the cycle since we're used to taking action in life. Think of it this way: move the body, and the mind will follow.

Yoga moves the body in specific ways to remove stored tension. This frees up energy from the fascia and muscular tissue and makes it available to be used in other ways (like creating new ways of thinking or being). Even the endorphins that kick in with movement put you in a better mood.

Yogic breathing also returns your awareness to the present moment. It's true that the subconscious mind sustains respiration without you having to think about it. Yet, you can use your conscious mind to shift the pattern of the breath on purpose. Specific exercises wake you up; others calm you down. The activity on page 102 helps you stay balanced amidst distractions.

Another way to directly change at the level of the body is to focus on gratitude. While you might think of this as a mental exercise, the body is the realm of emotions. Each cell stores emotional memory.[7,8] And your emotional state directly impacts your heart.

If you are stressed, te heart rhythm pattern is jagged and irregular, similar to that of an incoherent brain. When you cultivate feelings of appreciation, satisfaction, and love, the heart rhythm pattern moves into coherence. This leads to greater mental clarity and improved cognitive function.[9]

The New You

Once you have interrupted your old way of thinking and feeling, you liberate energy in the body. You free it up as raw material to create an exciting future.

You think in fresh ways. You perceive familiar circumstances from a new vantage point and fire neural networks differently. When you also shift your attitude from negative to positive, the brain is naturally recalibrated to a coherent state.

THE CYCLE OF POSITIVE CHANGE

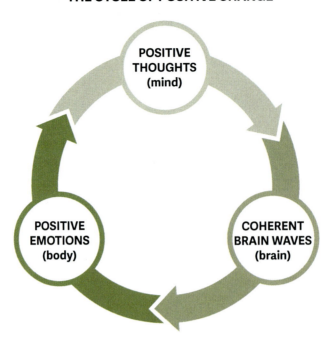

This is the headspace you're after on the course—one that is present, creative, and aligned with your golf goals.

A coherent brain then sends synchronized signals to the rest of the body. Your cardiovascular system, digestive system, immune system, and all systems can return to homeostasis. Instead of using your inner energy to survive, it can now be used for more productive reasons. You can focus on change and be excited about it.[10] A whole host of other life-affirming emotions, like appreciation and compassion, show up, too.

When you make changes at any one of these three areas, you live within a new cycle. With practice, positive thoughts become your new normal, creating coherent brain waves and a body fueled by harmony and supportive emotions. This becomes your new hamster wheel. Only instead of being tired and burned out after endless cycles, you're invigorated. You witness changes in yourself and in your golf game, and you're ready for more!

In the past, the conscious mind (5%) battled the subconscious (95%). Now, as the new you, they work together for your success.

And even if you do shank the ball or have an unlucky lie, you can retain a sense of humor. You can be open to interesting ideas and recover quickly. Chip Beck said it best when he would hit one into the woods, *"You gotta love it. This is what golf is all about."*

Activity: Flex the Muscles of Your Mind

This activity is a specific training plan to flex the muscles of your mind. If changing one belief is equivalent to one repetition, I suggest you complete three reps every day for the upcoming week. This solidifies each step in the mind, brain, and body. Here is the process:

Step 1: Identify the Negative Stress

The first step to change is to use your awareness and identify any stress in the mind. The easiest way to do this is to pinpoint negative beliefs. These are unwanted thoughts that get stuck on replay in your mind—ones that have become solidified as part of your belief system and identity. Ask yourself:
- What negative thoughts keep popping up regarding myself as a golfer or about my game specifically?
- Do I have any regrets?
- What are repeating problems in my game?
- What causes me to complain about my body? Or about my time on the course?

Write your ideas down in short, simple sentences. For example, you might write: *"I am anxious and tense when I hit out of the sand."* Or, *"My body is so stiff in cold weather, and I can't swing well."*

Numerous ideas might come to mind. I suggest only writing 1-3 statements for this activity. You can revisit the rest when you practice this exercise in the coming weeks ahead.

Step 2: Replace Negative with Positive

Now it's time to remove the weeds from your mental garden and plant new seeds instead. We'll do this by replacing the negative words with positive ones. To replace the negative word, think about its opposite.

Rather than being anxious or tense when hitting out of the sand, how might you want to be instead? You might prefer being confident, skilled, or graceful. Pick one and write a new sentence where the positive replaces the negative.

"I am ~~anxious~~ and ~~tense~~ when I hit out of the sand." ⟶ BECOMES ⟶ *"I am calm and confident as I hit out of the sand."*

Rather than being stiff when playing in the cold, how could your body be different? You might be strong, coordinated, or prepared. Write your new sentence as:

"My body is so ~~stiff~~ in cold weather, and I ~~can't swing well~~." → BECOMES → "My body is <u>strong</u> in cold weather, and I swing with <u>coordination</u>."

It's your turn to transform your negative sentences into positive ones. Don't worry if you don't believe these statements right away. This step only identifies how you want to be different. The actual shift will come in the next step.

Step 3: Internalize the New Belief

In Step 3, you transfer your statement from an idea in the conscious mind to a memorized belief of the subconscious. This is the re-programming phase. We'll do this by shifting your body posture, closing your eyes, and breathing deeply.

First, find a comfortable seated position. Cross one ankle over the other and then cross one wrist over the other. This position is known as a brain-integrated posture. Many yoga postures use crossover patterns because they noticed valuable effects as well. Basically, you're modifying the body to have a direct impact on the mind.

In a perfect world, the right and left hemispheres of your brain would work together effortlessly. Your left brain would analyze and decipher data from the

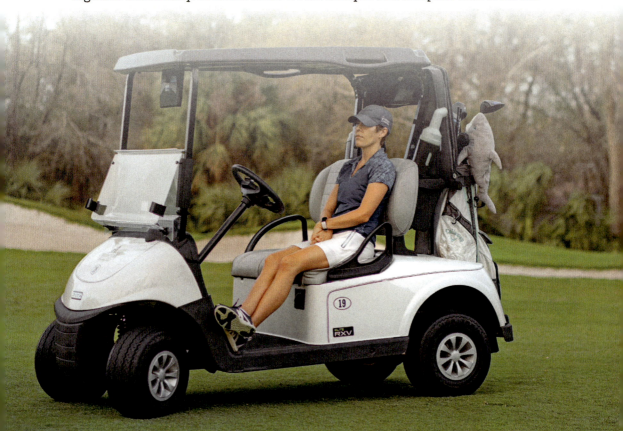

world around you. The right brain would understand these bits of data in relation to the bigger whole and make emotional sense of your experience. Yet one hemisphere tends to shut down in the face of stressful situations. That's why we use a brain-integrated state to restore communication between sides. This calms the mind, boosts memory, and creates a super learning state.

As you close your eyes, you remove external stimuli, and your brain waves move from beta to alpha. Slow down your breathing as you repeat your positive statement from Step 2. Select only one statement at a time. Continue to say this phrase to yourself until you get tired of saying it or notice an internal shift, which usually only takes 2-5 minutes. However, if you carry a lot of stress around the issue, it could take a bit longer.

As you finish, take a deep breath, and place your palms and fingertips to touch in Prayer Pose. This hand position is like hitting the save button on your mental computer.

> **TIP:** Prayer Pose is synonymous with Anjali Mudra (pronounced ahn-jah-lee moo-dra) in the yoga world. Anjali means *"offering"* in Sanskrit, and mudra means *"seal, mark, or sign."* No matter what you call it, this familiar gesture of drawing the hands together in front of the heart is a sign of respect. This might be directed toward others, as when greeting someone or saying goodbye. It can also be used to honor yourself as an integral part of the creative process.
>
>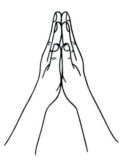
>
> We use Prayer Pose in this activity to indicate the right and left hemispheres of the brain are now aligned. It's also a symbol that you're blending the subconscious mind with the conscious one and linking inner changes with your outer ones.
>
> If you attend a yoga class, you'll often have a teacher end with Anjali Mudra and the phrase namaste (pronounced na-ma-stay). This Sanskrit word translates to *"the light within me bows to the light within you."* Essentially, it's a verbal way to appreciate the roles that both the student and teacher play in the learning experience.

Step 4: Create a Plan of Action

I agree with author John Maxwell that *"Understanding changes minds. Action changes lives."* Now that your belief is stored in the subconscious, it's time to take that new idea and put it into conscious action. To do this, select one activity you can do today to embody your new belief.

If your new statement is "I am calm and confident as to hit out of the sand," your action could be to schedule 30 minutes this week to practice sand shots. Or you could book a lesson with your golf pro. Maybe you even close your eyes for 5-10 minutes today and envision yourself hitting out of the bunker with ease.

If your sentence is *"My body is strong in cold weather, and I swing with coordination,"* you could integrate yoga into your pre-round warm-up (see page 74) to prepare your body on chilly days.

Every action you take is essentially a vote for the type of person and golfer you want to be.

The action plan you create helps you be that person now.

One final tip: Keep your action step simple and fun. Don't overcomplicate things or try too much at once! Think small wins, step-by-step, and these tiny wins add up to big victories over time!

Step 5: Celebrate!

In what way can you celebrate the success of flexing your mental muscles today? How can you honor the changes you're making in the mind?

Activity Summary: Flex the Muscles of Your Mind

Step 1: Identify negative self-talk
Write down a negative statement or feeling about yourself or your golf game. What negative self-talk is running through your brain?

Step 2: Eliminate the negative; replace it with a positive
Cross out the negative words from your sentence in step 1 and consider which positive ones could replace them. Rewrite a new positive sentence below and use the positive words sheet for suggestions as needed.

Step 3: Reprogram the new belief
It's time to write your new belief into the subconscious mind. Sit in a brain-integrated posture and breathe evenly. Then repeat your new, positive statement silently. When you're tired of saying your phrase to yourself, open your eyes and place your hands in namaste. Write down any insights you had during this step.

Step 4: Create a plan of action
What fun, clear action could you take today that would reinforce your positive statement from step 2?

Step 5: Celebrate!
In what way can you celebrate the success of flexing your mental muscles today? How can you honor the changes you're making in the mind?

Practice, Practice, Practice

James Clear, author of Atomic Habits, reminds us that *"Greatness is consistency. Meditating once is common. Meditating daily is rare. Exercising today is simple. Training every week is simply remarkable. Writing one essay rarely matters. Write every day, and you're practically a hero. Unheroic days can make for heroic decades."* [1]

When you flex your physical muscles at the gym, it takes 4-6 weeks to see a noticeable difference in the body. This is because changes are made at the subtle level first. The same goes for when you flex the muscles of your mind, like:

Learning new golf strategies and techniques. Visualizing your best round. Practicing gratitude. Getting on your yoga mat to move and breathe in deliberate ways.

Each of these techniques can stop the negative cycle that prevents your improvement. They also enhance your awareness and help you become a better golfer.

Yet these practices are just that—practices.

You want to repeat them consistently. You want them to become habits. Unlike a college degree which is permanently yours once the required courses are completed, personal alignment is not. Coherence isn't guaranteed from this moment forward. You'll need to be an active participant in the change process, and you'll want to attend to your mind, brain, and body so that they continue to function optimally.

As the great Arnold Palmer said, *"Success in this game depends less on strength of body than strength of mind and character."*

Putting it Together

Not only do you want to swing in a coordinated way on the course, but you also want to think efficiently, too. This requires that you first understand how the mind, brain, and body work together to make change happen. Then, you can remove unwanted mental debris. You can break negative cycles of thinking and playing, and you can flex the muscles of the mind to uplevel your game.

Take Action Now

- **Change your golf-related dialogue.**
  Complete the Flex the Muscles of Your Mind activity on page 61 three to five times this week. This rewires your perception, brain circuits, and body patterns to match your new mindset. And it should only take about 20-30 minutes of your time.

  Download a printable worksheet for this activity at www.TheFlexibleGolfer.com/free.

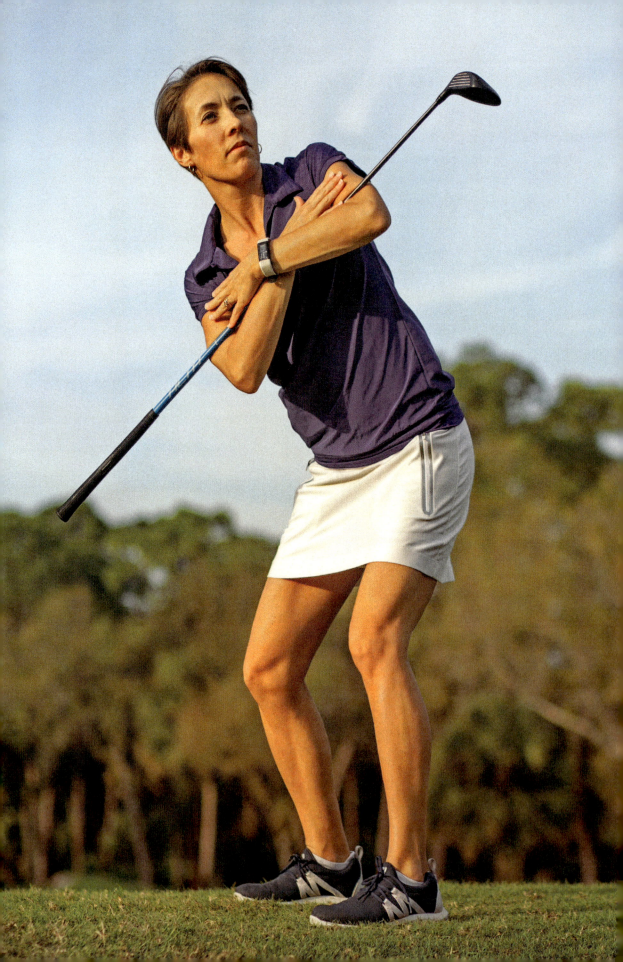

WEEK 3

Develop a Pre-Round Routine

"It's not the will to win that matters. Everyone has that. It's the will to prepare that matters."

–Paul "Bear" Bryant, football player and coach

WEEK 3 OVERVIEW

This week I'll let you in on my secret-weapon strategies that help me sustain high levels of energy and unwavering concentration on the course. This includes how to use your senses in an optimal way to remain calm and centered as you play.

Before we get into this week's material, I have a confession to make. A swarm of butterflies still take up residency in my belly each and every time I play golf with someone I don't know well. We might warm-up together on the range or putting green. They might tell me about their family and love for golf. I might even really like them and want to adopt them as my new best friend.

This doesn't cease the fluttering of those butterflies, though. They stick around for at least five holes.

If I didn't flex the muscles of my mind, this could ruin my game. I could appear inexperienced and sacrifice a few balls in the process. I could crumble and give up on my game.

Just like the professionals who remain composed under pressure, I, too, use the kaleidoscope of sensations in my body to enhance my focus. I channel it into deliberate actions before my round. I call this my pre-round routine, and it consists of mental and physical habits that prepare me to play well (no matter who I'm paired with).

When you select deliberate actions before your round, you set yourself to have the best round possible.

You also free up mental energy. As you discovered last week, your conscious mind has limited capacity. It can only process one to three events at a time. If you're frantically searching your bag for a ball mark or a last-minute snack, you can't pay attention to your golf game.

This week I'll reveal the most crucial elements of a pre-round routine. We'll address the importance of physically preparing the body for the golf swing. I'll show you the most common mental errors golfers make before they tee up and how to keep the fear of injury or a tragic mulligan on the first tee at bay. I'll also share some of my logistical go-to's that set me up for success on the course.

Benefits of a Pre-Round Routine

In case I haven't convinced you already, a pre-round routine has numerous benefits for your body and mind. A pre-round routine:

Provides purpose for your game. Whether you're out on the course to improve your score or have fun with your friends, a pre-round routine can highlight your reasons for playing. It also reinforces the kind of golfer you are and amplifies the fulfillment you experience on the course.

Creates a sense of calm. Maybe you don't get bombarded with butterflies before you play, yet you might experience a sense of anxiety or fatigue. This could be directly related to nerves about your game ahead, like in tournament settings. Or, you might have other life stressors that bleed into your time on the course. In any case, a pre-round routine can keep you grounded before play.

Fuels your energy and passion. Many sports teams use a pep talk or group chant to get them fired up before competition. Have you seen the Haka performed by New Zealand's All Blacks team? This ceremonial dance is enough to get me pumped up to play, and yet I don't want to go anywhere near a rugby field. Similarly, a pre-round routine is designed to get you excited to play, only not in the jittery, overly caffeinated kind of way. A pre-round routine trains you to be eager for your round without the hype that launches your cortisol levels into space. Instead, you can remain calm, eager, and aware.

Increases your awareness. Yes, a pre-round routine invites you to step back from the traditional knee-jerk responses we live by on a daily basis. You get to step into the role of a neutral observer. From this place, you make better decisions before you start the round and as you progress through it.

Boosts your confidence. With more awareness, you can tap into greater levels of confidence. You can trust your strategy and your swing, and you can remain poised during both easy and challenging shots alike.

Now that you understand the positive outcomes that arise from a pre-round routine, let's look at the different elements that comprise one.

You might already have a routine of your own in place. If this is the case, I suggest you cross-check your list with mine and refine yours to include each golf-ready element. If you don't have a plan already, the tips below will help you customize one now.

Elements of a Pre-Round Routine

A pre-round routine includes five basic elements. The goal is to keep your routine simple so you can memorize it and repeat it consistently. With more efficiency of your body and mind from the start, you free up energy to be creative and powerful on the course.

Element 1: Yoga

The first element of a pre-round routine involves general physical movement. As Dr. Craig Davis points out, *"The goal of any warm-up prior to golf or any sporting activity is the same: to move all necessary joints, associated muscles, and the connective tissue through a full range of motion in multiple planes of movement."*[1]

Yoga is one of the best ways you can do this. It lubricates the joints and enhances circulation. Yoga before a round of golf can also increase neurological activity and proprioception (body awareness), which leads to improved coordination from the start.

In a pre-round yoga routine, we start with the feet. Your feet anchor you to the ground, provide feedback about the surface beneath you, and initiate the golf swing. Once you boost sensations in the feet, we'll move up the kinetic chain to the hips. Many golfers develop lower back pain, or injury, because their hips aren't mobile or strong enough. If this is the case, the low back steps in during the swing to compensate. The exercises this week and in the cross-training classes on page 152 help prevent this.

Once we create stability and mobility in the hips, it's time to address the spine. We'll rotate the middle and upper thoracic spine to mirror the rotation needed for a powerful swing, and we'll engage the shoulder blades to support the shoulder girdle.

I've done these yoga poses regularly before my round, often next to my cart before our group tees off. Some of the ladies in my league gave me funny looks at first. Then once they read this book, and realized the value of each posture, they started doing some of them, too.

Not All Stretching is Created Equal

Before we explore the exact poses to get golf-ready, let me explain the types of stretching we'll use before your round. Research shows that not all stretching is created equal, and we want to stretch in ways that boost performance—not inhibit it.[2]

Dynamic Stretching: Also known as dynamic mobility, this style of stretching increases body temperature with fluid movements and is the best way to prepare for the powerful golf swing.[3,4] It improves your range of motion, speed, and agility.

Ballistic Mobility: This is a form of dynamic stretching where you bounce slightly in a pose near your end range of motion. Ballistic mobility hydrates the connective tissue and paves the way for greater range of motion.

Active Static Stretching: Static stretching refers to longer-held postures, and active means that some areas of the body contract to facilitate a stretch in other areas. The goal is to elongate and strengthen the muscular and connective tissues. To get the most benefit from active static stretching before golf, you'll only hold poses for less than 60-seconds.[5] We'll use this minimally in our pre-round routine and save more of it for cross-training between rounds (see week 6).

Now join me on the mat as I teach you how to apply these specific techniques in a pre-round yoga practice.

Activity: Pre-Round Yoga Practice

The postures below will ensure the major muscle groups and joints are warm before play. I suggest trying them out at home first. Then, as you are more comfortable with the movements, you can use them at the course, too.

Time: 20-30 minutes

1. Activate the Feet
Just as your feet initiate the backswing, you want awareness of your foundation to start your yoga warm-up. Use the exercise on page 30 to activate your feet first.

2. Half Sun Salute
The Sun Salutation is a foundational sequence in yoga as it combines a number of key postures. And just as the rising sun increases the Earth's temperatures, these poses build heat in the body. We'll take a modification known as a Half Sun Salutation:

3. Stabilize the Hips
Use the toe-tapping exercise on page 35 to turn on the hip stabilizers.

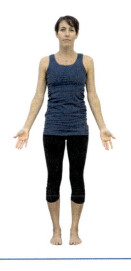

Stand in Mountain Pose with your hands by your side.

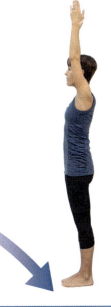

Inhale as you reach your arms into Upward Salute.

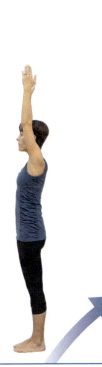

Inhale as you bring your torso and arms up into Upward Salute.

Half Sun Salute

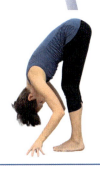

Exhale, as you move into a Standing Forward Fold.

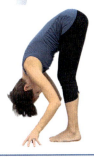

Exhale, and fold forward again. Bend the knees as needed.

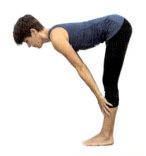

Inhale and lengthen the spine to come halfway up. Elongate your neck and gaze slightly forward.

DEVELOP A PRE-ROUND ROUTINE

4. Side Body Stretch

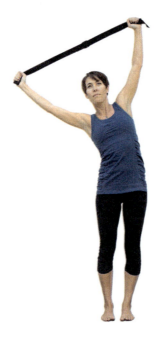

A side stretch targets many areas of the body used in the golf swing. You anchor down through the feet just like you do in your golf stance. Your spine remains neutral, and your core engages, and your torso also elongates. It's from this length you can effectively rotate the spine in your takeaway. Plus, you strengthen the arms by bringing them overhead.

Take a Side Bend
- As you inhale, reach both arms up overhead.
- Take your left hand and grab your right wrist. Then on your next exhale, lean to the left. As you near your maximum stretch, take 10-15 tiny bouncing movements with your torso. Then, hold still in the side stretch for 2-3 cycles of breath.
- Use your inhale to stand upright again. Switch the grip of your hands: your right hand grabs your left wrist. Then exhale as you bend to the right. Repeat the same actions on the other side.
- Inhale to come back to center. As you exhale, return your hands to your side, and take Mountain Pose once again.

You can also use a golf club or yoga strap for this posture as well. Just make sure that as you bend laterally, your head remains equally spaced between both arms.

5. Knee-to-Chest Movements

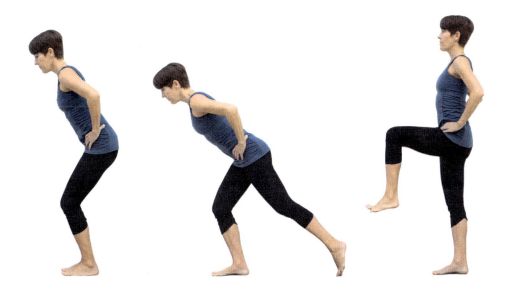

This dynamic activity builds strength in the outer hip muscles, which prepares the hips to remain stable as you swing your club. Begin in Chair Pose.

Toe Taps, then Knee-to-Chest
- Keep your hips level and steady, so there is as little movement as possible when you move.
- Transition your weight onto your left foot as you unweight the right. As you inhale, tap the toes of your right foot on the ground behind you. Reach back as far as possible without swaying the hips.
- Then press down through the left foot. Hug the left hip into the midline and bring the right knee toward the chest as you exhale.
- Repeat 5-15 times on this side, warming up the hip stabilizers on your left side. Then, repeat with your right foot grounded and your left leg in motion to warm up the right.

Rest in Mountain Pose when you are done. Observe any changes in the legs.

6. Standing Twist

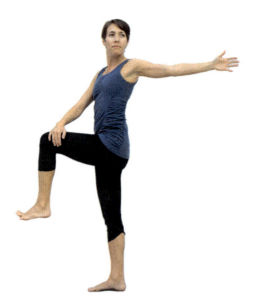

A strong core, which includes all the musculature around the midsection, protects the spine during a powerful golf swing. This pose will establish strength in the core and improve your balance simultaneously.

- Build a strong base of support with your left foot. Engage the left leg muscles and hip stabilizers by pressing into the ground. Draw your belly button in toward the spine. Relax your shoulders, jaw, and eyes as you hug your right knee into your chest.
- Find a point in front of you to gaze at.
- Stay in this simple balance. Or take your left hand to the outer edge of your right knee. Extend your right arm out to the side for additional balance. Imagine standing taller as your feet press down into the ground.
- Take 5-10 cycles of breath before switching to the other side.
- Stand with both feet on the ground momentarily before moving on to the next posture.

7. Crescent Lunge with a Side Stretch

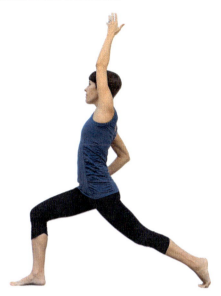

The Crescent Lunge Pose requires stability of the hips to remain balanced. When you add the side stretch, you give the body space from which to later twist during your golf swing.

Keep your feet hip distance apart and step your right foot forward 3-4 feet. Stay on the ball on your back foot. Bend your front knee generously until it is aligned over your front ankle (but no further). Draw your tailbone down as you lift your lower belly up. With your right hand on your hip, inhale to reach the left arm up overhead. Then, keeping your balance, slightly lean the torso to the right until you feel a slight stretch on the front of the left thigh and/or left side of the body. Hold for 5-8 rounds of breath. Then, reverse your steps to come out of the pose and move to the other side.

8. Mobilize the Shoulder Blades

Moving further up the body, it's time to bring more movement to the shoulder blades specifically. Revisit the yoga movements from page 42 to get your shoulders ready to play. Alternate between Cactus Arms and Eagle Arms 5-10 times.

9. Skater Pose

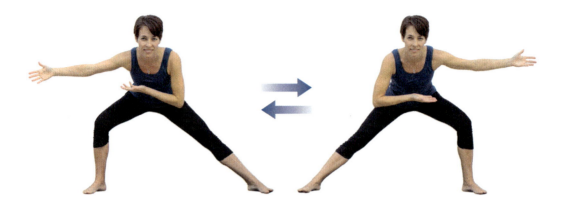

Turn to the side of the mat and take your legs wide. You've prepared the outer hips for stability up to this point. It's now time to strengthen and elongate the inner thighs.

- Turn your heels in and toes out. Sink your hips down like you would sit into a Chair Pose. Look down to make sure your toes and knees point out at the same angle.Slowly shift your weight side-to-side. As the weight moves to your right leg, straighten your left (and vice versa).
- Repeat 5-10 times on each side.
- Then, hold Skater Pose with your right knee bent. Find your end range of motion where you can still breathe deeply. Pulse slightly 10-15 times, then hold still for 2-3 rounds of breath. Repeat this ballistic mobility and static stretching technique on the second side.

10. Wide-Legged Forward Fold

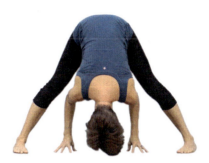

It's time to elongate the back of the body, including the inner hamstrings, in a Wide-Legged Forward Fold. Stay facing the side of your mat. With the legs straight and your pelvis neutral, turn your toes slightly inward toward the midline. This slight internal rotation at the hip mirrors what is needed in your backswing.

Keep your hands on your hips for balance. Inhale to lengthen the spine and keep your collarbones broad. Exhale and fold forward. Stay for 8-10 cycles of breath. Place your hands anywhere on the floor or props for support.

To come out, exhale and bring your hands to your hips first. Draw your belly button toward the spine and use the inhale to return the torso all the way upright.

11. Twisted Chair, Golfer Variation

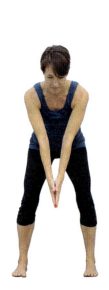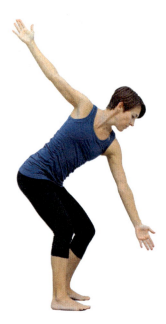

Your legs are warm, and your spine is mobile. Now you're going to take a practical movement similar to the golf swing—one in which the hips and shoulders work together. Better still, your torso hinging forward requires your core to engage. This protects your spine as you move on the mat and the course.

- Set your feet similar to your golf stance. Bring your palms together at the midline with the arms dangling naturally in front of you. Activate your feet, legs, and core.
- As you exhale, shift to the inner edge of your right foot as you twist to the right and extend your right arm up. Inhale to come back to center. Exhale and twist to the left, bringing your weight to the inner edge of your left foot as you twist the hips, spine, and arm to the left.
- Repeat 5-15 times on each side.

12. Mountain Pose

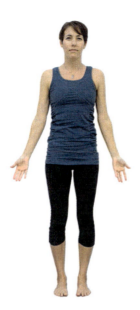

Finish your pre-golf warm-up the same way you started—in a symmetrical Mountain Pose. Breathe deeply here for at least one minute. By pausing in stillness, you can sense the changes in your body. You're more balanced, stable, and strong. You can tap into the clarity of your mind as well. Mostly, you reinforce that you're ready to play your best as you step up to the first tee box in your game.

Element 2: Golf-Specific Warm Up

Yoga awakens the body in a general sense. Now it's time to actually swing your golf clubs and get ready with the golf-specific actions you'll repeat on the course. Remember, the goal with a pre-round routine is to have habits you can repeat easily and consistently. You want to select golf-specific drills that are the same, freeing up mental energy to focus on the nuances of the day.

Here are the logistics of my golf warm-up:

First, I visit the putting green. Since this club will be the one I use most throughout the round, I want to get familiar with it early. I want to get a distinct feel of the greens. To do this, I practice:

- 15-foot putts on a level surface toward the fringe. This takes the idea of the cup out of the equation at first.
- 20- and 30-foot putts uphill and downhill to gauge speed. Most times, I aim for a spot on the green first, then I focus on a specific hole.
- 6- to 8-foot putts from a variety of lies.
- 2- to 3-foot putts last, to memorize the sound of my ball sinking into the cup.

Then, I move to the chipping area and work with a few distances and types of shots. From there, I visit the range to hit balls with my 7-iron, 5-hybrid, and driver. Since our local course requires a driver from the first tee, I end my time on the range with that specific swing. This embeds a great shot in my body and mind right before stepping up to the tee box.

This entire golf warm-up can last 45-60 minutes. If I arrive at the course early, I enjoy this leisurely practice session before play. Yet, if I only have 20-30 minutes before our tee time, I'll still follow the exact same routine (only I spend less time with each club).

While this golf warm-up works for me, I recognize it might not be right for you. I suggest you create your own logical sequence of golf-specific drills to use repeatedly before each round.

> **TIP:** There are days I get delayed with work and don't have time to visit the range at all. That's why I keep a 3-pack of Wiffle balls in my golf bag. I can stand in the practice area and simulate my full swing with a tangible object, which heightens the eye-hand coordination I'll need from the very first moment of the game.

Element 3: Set an Intention

This component of your pre-round routine can take very little time. It's where you set an intention for the upcoming round. As Dr. Joe Dispenza says, *"An intention is getting clear about what you want. That's it!"*

The yogic sages of India knew the value of this thousands of years ago. They understood that our intentions ultimately shape our future. So, when you set an intention for your golf game now, you set the tone of what's to come before any action takes place.

On a simple level, an intention is a thought or group of thoughts about how you want things to be in your experience, and those thoughts send signals to your body and your environment as a result.

Intentions can be general thoughts that result from your wide array of life experiences. These pop up naturally and continually throughout your day. For example, if someone is mean to you, you want to interact with others in a more kind and compassionate way. If you are misunderstood, you seek understanding. Or, if you get injured, then you set an intention to be well once again.

Your intentions before golf, though, will likely be very specific in nature. You might set an intention to:

- Be more lighthearted during your round
- Speak nicer to yourself after a bad shot
- Stand tall throughout the round to reinforce your confident play
- Complete a full breath out before stepping up to the ball
- Remember your single swing thought before your takeaway

If you're new to the idea of setting an intention, I suggest you do the following:

Find a quiet space before your round. This could be an extra moment in your car alone before you step out to meet your foursome. Or you might savor a few minutes in the cart by yourself while your partner finishes up on the range.

Then ask yourself, *"What would it be like if _____ ?"* (and fill in the blank). For example:

- What would it be like if I felt steady in my swing today?
- What would it be like if I hit my drives straight, or I had a smooth putting stroke?
- What would it be like if I only focused on my good shots and put the wild ones behind me?

Your ability to ask *"What if"* questions opens your mind to the possibilities of new outcomes. You also release the need to know how those outcomes will play out during your round. This keeps you more relaxed before, and during, play.

Finally, close your eyes and imagine your *"What if"* situation playing out over the next few hours. Engage as many of your senses as possible to do this. Notice what physical sensations would be present in the body. Imagine what you would hear others say or what you would say to yourself. Paint a picture of what your intention would look like as well.

This naturally leads to the next element of your pre-round routine: visualization.

Element 4: Visualize Your Round

Jack Nicklaus is famous for saying: *"I never hit a shot, not even in practice, without having a very sharp in-focus picture of it in my head."*

Nicklaus, like many athletes today, understood the power of visualization. Visualization is a great tool to imagine your future experience. You have about 11 million sensory receptors in the body, and ten million of those are dedicated to the eyes alone. This is why identifying what you want to see during your round is important. You can imagine how high your ball would fly in the air, how it would land and roll out toward the green, and even see the ball dropping into the cup.

What's amazing is that research today reveals your body can actually change just by your thoughts alone. In one study, subjects were asked to do 60-minutes of finger exercises against resistance over the course of 4 weeks. The result? A 30% increase in muscle strength. Not anything to get excited about, I know. However, a second group mentally practiced the same activity without ever lifting a finger, and they gained a 22% increase in muscle strength.[6] This study, as well as others since, demonstrate that the body and brain changed without physical exertion.[7,8]

You can prime your body for a strong, consistent golf swing before you pick up your clubs, too. And you can help your body memorize any intention before your round with your imagination alone.

I suggest pairing this visualization element of your pre-round routine with that of setting an intention. You're already in a quiet space so you can focus. Plus, you can have something to focus on—whether that be a specific aspect of your game or an attribute you wish to embody throughout the round.

You can continue to practice the skill of visualization as you approach each new hole on the course. I suggest incorporating it into your pre-shot routine (see page 104). Remember, the more you use this skill, the more hardwired it gets in the brain and supports your positive cycle of change.

Element 5: Double-Check Your Supplies

Now that your body and mind are primed for play, it's time to double-check your supplies for the round. I call this my comfort kit. Just like you would make sure you were well-stocked before going on a long hike, weekend camping trip, or long road trip, you want to do the same before departing the clubhouse.

A lot can happen in a 4-hour round. The weather can change. Your energy levels fluctuate. When you create a comfort kit, you ensure your basic needs can be met on the course. You won't find yourself scrambling to organize logistics before the starter calls your name. And, you can use the extra mental bandwidth on other details of the day that could affect your game.

Your comfort kit might include:
- Water
- Snacks
- Sunscreen
- Chapstick
- Sunglasses cleaner
- Kleenex or napkins
- Extra layers of clothing
- GPS device and charger
- Cell phone and charger
- Extra cash

The options are endless. Just think of which situations could create a distraction during the round and use your comfort kit to prevent that from happening. Even a small first aid kit can be useful to store in your bag. During a recent tournament, one of my teammates unexpectedly cut her finger. Only one member in our foursome was prepared with a Band-Aid. Because of her, we were able to immediately cover the wound and swing our way to victory without ever missing a beat.

You can add more items for sheer enjoyment, too. My 85-year-old friend carries a fifth of Fireball for celebratory moments. Another installed a clown horn on her cart for the same reason.

Have fun as you pack the items for your round that will sustain your focus and keep your spirits high. You can use the checklist on the next page to jot down your ideas.

Pre-Round Checklist

This checklist will cover the items you can include in your pre-round routine. This will ensure you are as prepared as possible to start your game.

Yoga Practice (20-30 minutes):
If you take the time just before your round to do yoga, you can warm up the tissues and prepare the body for the powerful swinging movements to come.
- ☐ General yoga practice

Golf Warm-Up (15-60 minutes):
Now that the body is warm in the general sense, it's time to dedicate some attention to golf-specific skills. Ensure that you take a few minutes for each of these aspects of your game (if possible).
- ☐ Putting
- ☐ Chipping/ Wedge
- ☐ Irons
- ☐ Driver

Intention Setting (5-10 minutes):
Set a clear focus for your game from the beginning to be more confident as you play.
- ☐ Write your intention on your scorecard

Visualize Your Round (5-10 minutes):
The goal is to use your senses to see, hear, and embody your intention.
- ☐ Close your eyes for a few minutes and imagine highlights of your round ahead

Double-Check Your Supplies (5-15 minutes):
Set yourself up for success by having the right things packed and with you when you play.
- ☐ Water
- ☐ Snacks
- ☐ Sunscreen
- ☐ Chapstick
- ☐ Sunglasses / Sunglass cleaner and cloth
- ☐ GPS and charger
- ☐ Cell phone and charger
- ☐ _____
- ☐ _____
- ☐ _____
- ☐ _____

Putting it Together

A pre-round routine gives structure to the time before your round. This way, you can prepare the body and mind in the most orderly way possible. Specific yoga poses, setting an intention, and a comfort kit are all part of this process. Then, with all the extra energy you save with your routine, you can focus on the unique elements of the day and adjust accordingly.

Take Action Now

- ❏ **Do yoga.**
  Get on your mat and try this week's yoga poses at home. When you are confident in the movements, you can take them to the course and use them before your round.

- ❏ **Prepare before your round.**
  Create your own comfort kit and ensure your bag is well-stocked before your next tee time.

You can take a simple pre-round yoga class with me and download a copy of this checklist at TheFlexibleGolfer.com/free.

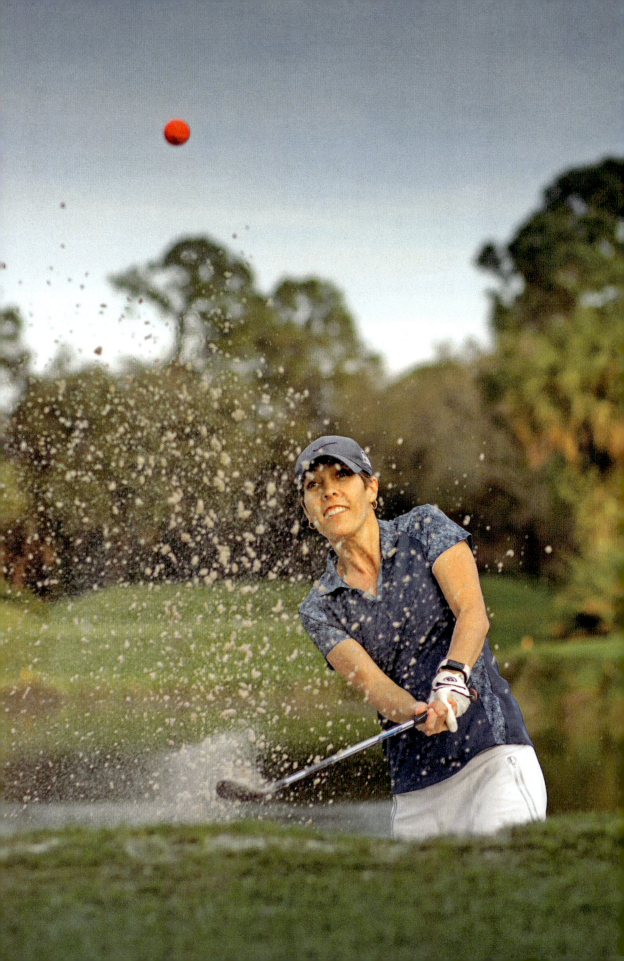

WEEK 4

Conserve Energy on the Course

"I used to resent obstacles along the path, thinking 'If only that hadn't happened, life would be so good.' Then I suddenly realized, life is the obstacles. There is no underlying path. Our role is to get better at navigating those obstacles. I strive to find calm, measured responses and to see hindrances as a chance to problem-solve."

—Janna Levin, physics and astronomy professor [1]

WEEK 4 OVERVIEW

You've done the work to prepare your body and mind for your round. Now it's time to keep that positive momentum going on the course. You do this by managing your energy efficiently. But how? This week, you'll discover ways in which a steady gaze, deliberate breath, and organized pre-shot routine can sustain a higher level of performance, and enjoyment, as a golfer.

During the editing process of this week's material, a golf joke kept coming to mind. It goes like this:

Kevin showed up at his office Monday morning and looked absolutely exhausted. His workmate, Claire, noticed right away. *"Kevin. You look terrible. Are you okay?"*

Kevin replied, *"Oh my gosh! Yesterday was a sad and difficult day."*

"What happened?"

"Well, you know I have a standing tee time with my friends each Sunday. Yesterday on the fifth hole, my playing partner, Charlie, had a heart attack and died."

"Oh, that's awful!" Claire sympathized. *"I am so sorry to hear that. It must have been horrible."*

"It was! For the whole rest of the game, it was hit the ball, drag Charlie. Hit the ball, drag Charlie."

This joke tickles my funny bone for two reasons.

First, golfers are a dedicated group. I love your commitment to the game, and I imagine your devotion rivals that of Kevin's (although I am glad you don't have to carry the corpse of a dearly departed companion twelve holes to prove it).

The reality is we often tow invisible baggage around the course with us. It might not fit in a body bag, but it's just as heavy and energetically draining. It's as though the joke's not about Kevin at all. It's about us, and how we make the game of golf more difficult than it already is. This is the second reason I always smile when I hear this story.

This week, I'll point out common challenges you face in golf. You could encounter cold temperatures and windy conditions. You might be tired due to a poor night's rest or distracted about the houseguests set to arrive tomorrow. Or you just might feel out of sync with your swing.

These inner and outer obstacles may always exist. Yet if you learn how to focus, you can mitigate unwanted effects of such challenges and pivot at any time during your game to get back on track.

Challenges of the Golf Game

Let's start with the most obvious reasons golf demands your full attention to play well.

The Ball is Stationary

Golf is different from most sports in that you encounter the ball in a stationary position.

The ball is not hurling toward you, like a baseball batter receiving a pitch or a tennis player about to return a serve. In golf, the ball just sits there. It simply waits for you to step up and hit it.

This is difficult because it's far more natural for your body to react to an object in motion. You move instinctively in those moments. But because you're not required to make a split-second decision about your swing, you can analyze and overanalyze each shot.

Your conscious mind searches its memory bank for useful information. It also assesses potential outcomes of a chosen line or club selection. These thoughts become like a pinball that ricochets between the past and future, landing anywhere but the present moment.

In this disconnected state, you lose trust in yourself and your swing. You can also overlook possibilities when you're not thinking clearly. The strategies this week will train your mind back into a focused, intuitive state—one in which you can confidently stand over a stationary ball and execute the skills you honed during practice.

There is a Time-Lapse Between Shots

There is a large time-lapse between each shot on the golf course. In other sports, you must actively pay attention to what's going on across the field or on the court even when you're not directly involved in the play. Not in golf. You can mentally check-out for minutes on end.

This time-lapse can lead to negative side effects.

The first is that you think about your upcoming shot long before you stand over the ball. You fret about the lie or the angle into the green. Or you get excited that your ball is nestled so close to the hole you can practically hear the birdie calling your name. This wastes mental energy too soon during your round.

Second, you can easily let your mind wander when you're not up to hit. You might chat with your friends, check your Facebook status, or review your NFL fantasy team standings. These actions might not affect you *if* you can return your attention back to the game. Many times, though, you can't. Your body continues to go through the motions, yet your mind is somewhere else entirely. A less-than-optimal score is often the result.

The trick to staying focused during this time-lapse is to train your mind like you do your muscles. We use yoga to activate specific muscles when they're needed, and fully relax them when not. When you do this with your thoughts, the time between shots can be a productive space to regroup. It can also amplify your enjoyment on a beautiful course. We'll explore specific ways to do this in a minute.

You're Responsible for Each Decision

Another challenge in golf is that you, alone, are responsible for your shots. It's just you and your ball out there. One shot you take directly impacts the lie for your next shot, which isn't a problem when you're hitting the ball well. In those streaks, you probably give yourself a hearty (yet invisible) pat on the back.

Only, you have no one else to blame when things go awry.

I'm the oldest of four kids in my family, so I always had a scapegoat when things went wrong during playtime. This is true in collaborative sports, too. Let's say you're a quarterback who throws a perfect spiral to a receiver in the endzone, and they drop the ball. Sure, you'd probably be disappointed. But deep down, you would remember the incomplete pass wasn't your fault.

In golf, you can try to blame a hosel rocket on a cell phone ringing unexpectedly or a gust of wind blowing hair in your face. You can complain that the course is too wet or too dry; the greens are too fast or too slow. You and I both know it's easier to attribute our mistakes to something outside of ourselves. It's far more satisfying to direct our anger or frustration elsewhere.

What likely happens, though, is you turn the finger of blame on yourself. You might verbally express your dissatisfaction with a shot, or you internally criticize your skills. This might even create a downward spiral of negativity that taints any future shot and prevents any possibility of mental recovery.

> **NOTE:** When you experience blame, frustration or anger on the golf course, your sympathetic nervous system turns on, heightening your focus short-term. However, it diminishes your health in the long run. That's why we'll use recovery techniques in week 5 to balance the body and mind after your round.

Thankfully, this doesn't have to be your story on the course. You can flex the muscles of your mind, like we did last week, and remain lighthearted in the face of such responsibility. Better still, you develop the mental resilience to recover quickly should an errant shot arise.

Your Score is Easy to Calculate

Your golf score is easy to calculate and easy to access during every round. This isn't a problem if you have a healthy relationship with the numbers you see on your scorecard. By this, I mean you view your score as a neutral feedback mechanism. Your score reflects how well the systems you have in place as a golfer, like your pre-shot routine, are working for you on any given day. Your score can also be used to track your progress and highlight deficiencies in your game.

However, problems arise when your thoughts and emotions fluctuate in direct correlation to your score. Many golfers rate their overall experience on the course based on their scorecard. If the numbers are low, they feel great about their round. If the scores are high, they don't. And if the numbers are close to hitting a personal record during a round, the pressure to perform well on each shot amplifies tremendously. These highs and lows ultimately drain your energy.

Yoga teaches you to view these fluctuations with a neutral eye instead. You'll learn how to shift your focus away from uncontrollable outcomes and back to the present moment. As you do this, the score will take care of itself.

Focus is a Skill

To overcome each of these challenges, you want to improve your mental focus. According to the Merriam-Webster dictionary, focus is how you direct your attention, and it's a state of clarity.[2] A growing body of scientific research also shows that focus is a skill.[3] This means it's more than an automatic response. Focus is a talent you can acquire and refine with practice.

Just as when you learn any other skill, you start with the basics. Then, through repetition, you internalize those behaviors as habits.

Let's start with a fundamental principle of focus.

Concentration is like a light switch. You can turn it on when attention is needed in your game and turn it off when it's not. In both settings, your focus remains in the present moment, which is your source of sustained energy throughout your round.

So, when do you *turn on* your concentration as a golfer?

I propose you narrow your focus in moments that directly impact your performance. This includes, but is not limited to, when you:

- Assess the lie of your ball
- Analyze an upcoming shot
- Use specific systems to execute your skills, like a pre-shot routine (which we'll cover on page 104)
- Take your swing
- Interpret internal cues that relate to your well-being, like hunger or thirst
- Reflect on your overarching intention(s) for playing golf

By training yourself to be a mindful golfer, you deliberately turn on your concentration. You learn to pay more attention to what's happening and what you're doing to create a better outcome on the course. Studies show that being more mindful changes the gray matter in your brain and improves body awareness.[4] It also boosts self-acceptance.[5] The result is a greater trust in your capabilities and the freedom to let go of the past.

Now, when do you *turn off* your concentration?

The goal is to broaden your focus once a critical decision has been made for your game. You want to do this when:

- Other people are hitting
- You're walking or driving to your ball
- You are waiting on the group ahead of you

Remember, staying present is what's most important. The techniques we'll explore now teach you to do this in simple, yet powerful, ways. I suggest you read through each method first. Then, decide on one or two you'd like to practice this week.

Select a Gazing Point

The first technique you can tap into regularly on the course is finding a dristi. A dristi is known in Sanskrit as a gazing point, and dristana is the practice of holding your focus on that point.

Your gaze is important because there are approximately 10 million sensory receptors in the eyes alone, and the mind tends to follow what you're looking at. You tend to focus on what you see. A dristi taps into this visual power and directs your attention into the present moment.

In a yoga practice, we use several dristi. You can stare off the tip of your nose. You can gaze past your fingertips. You watch the dancing flame of a candle during an eyes-open meditation.

Turn on Focus with Your Gaze

On the golf course, you can use a dristi to stay aware of what matters most. Turn on your concentration by looking at the target where you want your ball to land or at the location where you want the ball to stop. You can even pinpoint the exact spot on the cup you want the ball to hit as it drops into it. The more specific, the better!

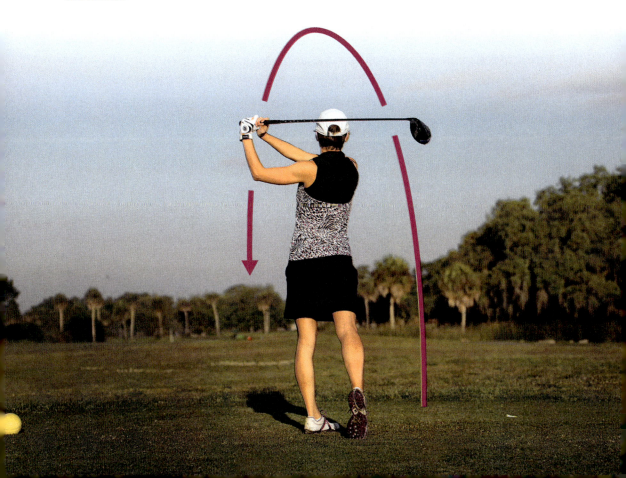

I keep a shark club head cover on my 3-wood as a visual cue that it's time to flip my focus into the "on" position. This plush great white is there each and every time I select a club, and just by looking at it, I'm reminded to be fierce and diligent with my attention. You could have a distinct bag tag or lucky charm that serves the same purpose.

While there are endless options to use as your dristi on the golf course, I suggest you select gazing points that are most meaningful to you.

Turn Off Focus with a Different Focal Point

When it's time to switch your focus into the "off" position, select a new dristi—one that is unrelated to your game. You could stare up at the puffy, white clouds and watch them float across the sky. You might observe other elements of nature, such as a nearby bird constructing a nest or a cottontail rabbit nibbling on grass. You might watch the shot of your playing partner and cheer on their success. Even the clear water in your bottle could capture your attention.

Your focus follows your gaze. Take note of what you see during your round, and use your eyes to make your golf day the most delightful experience possible.

Use a Mantra

A mantra is a sound, word, or phrase that draws your attention into the moment. The word mantra can be broken down into two parts—'Man,' which means mind and 'tra' which means transport. Thus, a mantra is the vehicle by which you regain focus. It heightens your awareness. And a mantra is repeated in a yoga practice to transcend the busyness of the mind.

The most common one is OM, or AUM, which is associated with the essential sound of the universe or the originating sound of creation. Another familiar mantra in yoga is So Hum. This mantra translates to *"I am that,"* and helps you identify with the infinite nature of your being.

The wonderful book, *The Legend of Bagger Vance*, entertains this idea.[6]

O.B. Keeler, a reporter, asks Bagger Vance, *"Are you equating the swing with the soul, the Authentic Soul?"*

"I prefer the word Self," Bagger Vance said. *"The Authentic Self. I believe this is the reason for the endless fascination of golf. The game is a metaphor for the soul's search for its true ground and identity."*

A mantra helps connect with your Authentic Self as you turn your focus on. You can repeat a word like *"breathe,"* or *"focus,"* or *"steady"* as you concentrate on your game.

Then, when you want to remain present between shots, you might create a longer mantra. My favorite: *"As I connect with Divine, I score pars and birdies on the back nine."* My goal with this phrase is to keep my energy high until the very last shot of my game.

Whether you're using a mantra to turn on your concentration or to turn it off, I recommend that you write your mantra on your scorecard. This adds visual power to your words and helps you naturally tune out distractions that could lower your energy.

Point Out the Obvious

You can also fine-tune your focus through the point-and-call technique used in the Japanese railway system for safety and efficiency. Steve and I use it each night to ensure all checklist items at home are buttoned up before bed.

The method is this: point at an object of importance and speak aloud what you see.

For example, I go through the house each evening and say aloud, *"The front door is locked. The side door is locked. The thermostat is set. The dog's been out. The coffee pot is on."*

This may sound redundant and boring. However, when something becomes a habit in your life, your comfort level increases. You become less sensitive to feedback. You get used to doing what you've always done, so your body and brain assume things will be the same in the future.

Only this energy-saving mechanism is not efficient on the golf course because every shot *is* different. Every shot *is* new. You need a heightened sense of awareness to address the uniqueness of each moment. You want a sharp focus.

Turn On Your Concentration

You can do this throughout your round by pointing-and-calling what you see. You might look at your ball and say, *"My ball is in thick grass."* You might assess the stance and say, *"The ball is uphill of my feet."* You can look at the flag and say, *"The pin is at the back of the green."*

I often state my intentions, such as, *"My aim is 10 yards left of the hole to account for the wind."* If we're ever paired together, don't be surprised if I lean over and share my thoughts out loud with you.

The words you speak become the verbal cues that increase your focus. They also prevent errors, enhance your creativity, and add more clarity to any situation you encounter during your game.

Assume a Brain-Integrated Posture

While the point-and-call technique helps you turn on your concentration, the brain-integrated posture is a way to turn it off. This pose broadens your perspective and neutralizes your energy.

We used it in week 2 as a way to change beliefs at the core of your being (see page 62). Now we can apply it in another capacity to stay present on the golf course.

Here's how it works. When you establish a crossover pattern with the body, more information is shared between both hemispheres of the brain. The quality of communication between the two sides increases as well.[7]

I treasure the brain-integrated posture because it reduces stress before taking a difficult shot. And since it's a discreet body position, nobody else knows what I'm doing. I simply look like I'm relaxing in my golf cart while my partner hits their ball.

Breathe On Purpose

Breathing on purpose is one of the best ways to stay present on the golf course. As you focus on your breathing, you get rid of tension and prevent unwanted distractions from interfering with your own game.

Like the brain-integrated posture, it's also simple to integrate into your round. Before we get into specific breathing exercises (called Pranayama), let's review the four parts of the breath.

The Inhale: The diaphragm contracts and descends, which allows the lungs to fill with air. When breathing deeply, you can feel the rib cage and belly expand due to your inhale.

The Pause After the Inhale: This pause will occur naturally, but you can also consciously pause here and hold this phase of the breath to increase clarity in the mind.

The Exhale: As you breathe out, the diaphragm relaxes and lifts in this phase, causing the lungs to expel any air within them. You can breathe out naturally, calmly and smoothly. Or you can create a more forceful exhalation, such as what happens when you blow out a candle. In this latter form, you're engaging more abdominal and intercostal muscles to do so.

The Pause After the Exhale: There is a natural pause that occurs before you inhale again. You can also hold the breath out on purpose, leaving the lungs temporarily empty. Just make sure you don't experience physical or mental strain as you do this, though.

Conscious breathing, like focus, is a skill. It takes time and repetition to get comfortable with these components of respiration. This box breathing activity will help you do just that. Before we start it, though, I want to show you how the breath can influence your attention.

Turn On Your Concentration With the Breath
When I prepare for a shot, I take a few deep cycles of breath. Then, I focus on taking a slow, full outbreath before stepping up to the ball. This is the "O" in PIVOT on page 105.

Turn Off Your Concentration, and Stay Present with Box Breathing
The box breathing techniques below return your power to the present moment. You successfully shift your attention away from details of your game to those of your breath.

Activity: Box Breathing

This activity interrupts your natural breathing pattern to enhance your attention.

Step 1: Get Grounded
The first step in this process is to get grounded. Said another way, it's time to tell your body and mind you're about to do something important. Take a very deep, deliberate breath or tune into sensations on the soles of your feet.

Step 2: Change Your Breathing Pattern
Now you're going to alter the pattern of your breathing on purpose. We'll use the shape of a box as the visual anchor for this process. Each segment of your breath will correspond to one side of the box, and you can trace the rectangle or square on your scorecard as you complete each segment. Select one of the two options below:

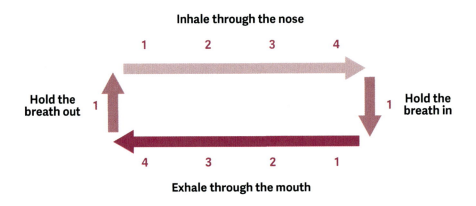

2A. On your inhale, count how long it takes you to breathe in. That equates to the top line of your rectangle. Then hold the breath in for a count of 1. Match the length of your exhale to the length of your inhale. Then hold the breath out for a count of 1. Repeat this entire process 3-5 more times.

Your breathing pattern might look like the box pictured above. If your count is slightly different, that's okay. Just stay as relaxed as possible while you breathe. Avoid forcing the breath in a way that creates tension in the body.

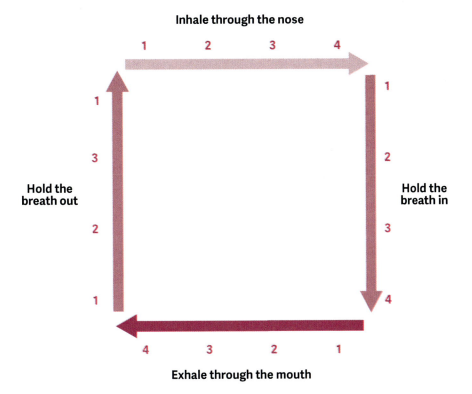

2B. This second box breathing technique matches all four segments of the breath to the same count. Count how long it takes you to breathe in. Hold the breath in for the same count. Then exhale to the same count. Hold the breath out for the same count, too. Repeat your conscious breathing technique 3-5 times around your box.

Step 3: Return to Your Natural Breathing Pattern
Allow your breath to flow naturally once again.

Step 4: Observe the Effects
Pause for a moment. Notice the immediate effects on your body and mind. Does your body appear lighter? Is your mind clearer? Do you notice any other shifts as a result of your intentional breathwork?

Step 5: Return to Your Game with Greater Awareness
You've still got more of your game to play. Do so with greater presence, clarity, and awareness, and revisit this activity anytime to focus back into the present moment.

PIVOT with Your Pre-Shot Routine

A pre-shot routine helps the mind and body align as one when you step up to swing. The pre-shot routine is where you prepare, analyze, and mentally rehearse your shot. You pair an elevated emotion (like remembering your best swing or best shot of the past) and pair it with the logical mind. It's from this structure in your game that you save energy and can turn your focus to the nuances of each shot.

Practice Swing

A practice swing transfers ideas from the thinking mind into the body. It helps me assess the ground beneath my feet, the stance I'll need to take to stay balanced during my swing, and any changes that will need to be made to my swing based on the lie and direction of my desired shot. The practice swing incorporates all these details at the level of the subconscious mind to use when you step up to hit. And it provides even more information from which to set an intention.

Intention

An intention is simply how you want things to be. You set the broad aim for your round before starting play (see -insert page) Now, it's time to create a specific intention for your next shot. It's time to craft a plan for your upcoming hit. To do this, ask yourself the following questions:
- What type of shot do I want to take?
- What distance do I want the ball to fly in the air?
- How far do I want it to roll out once it lands?
- What risks affect this type of shot?
- Are there environmental factors to consider, like wind or rain?
- Are there rewards that will outweigh the risks?

Trust the answers that come instinctively. Then, from this clear-minded perspective, it's time to mentally rehearse your shot.

Visualization

Visualization uses your imagination to mentally rehearse your upcoming swing and ball movement. Research shows that the mind responds in the same way when the eyes witness an event externally and when you imagine something internally. Envision the best shot possible before you hit the ball. Tap into your reservoir of past knowledge and remember what a coordinated swing feels like. Hear the perfect ping echoing off your club. Listen to the ball dropping into the hole. The more senses you bring on board in this process, the more real it becomes at the level of the subconscious mind.

Outbreath

Many people miss-hit their golf shots because tension still exists in their mind and body. When you take a purposeful outbreath, you signal to your mind that it's time to chill out. Your body knows how to swing, and a deep breath out reinforces that you're ready to have your body work its magic.

As B.K.S. Iyengar, a leader in the yoga industry says, the exhalation is *"The process by which the energy of the body gradually unites with that of the mind."* You want this unity when you step up to the ball. A deep outbreath—slow and through the mouth—will help you achieve this.

Trust Your Swing

As you start to walk forward toward your ball, it's essential to embrace the trust you have in yourself. You want to have a level of faith that your body can execute the picture you created with the mind.

The previous steps in the PIVOT process build inner alignment. The practice swing gives your body immediate feedback so it can make subtle changes and adapt for the unique shot at hand. Your intention then clarifies the mind, so you intellectually understand the goal. The visualization element brings all your senses on board, and the outbreath is a final reminder that you've got this. So, smile and step up to swing with confidence.

Move the Body

Just as yoga postures prepare your body to play golf, they can be used on the course to stay mobile, warm, and energized throughout the round.

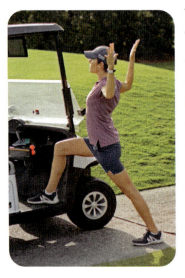

Warrior 1

This standing pose stretches the calves, hip flexors, and shoulders. It's also a great way to keep your hips warm and mobile for your golf swing. Start in Mountain Pose. Step your right foot forward, just longer than a walking step. Your right toes will point forward. Your left foot will turn out slightly. Bend your front knee until it aligns over your ankle. Continue to press down through the outer edge of your back foot as you lift your arms up. You can reach straight up or take Cactus Arms to open the chest. Keep your hips and torso pointing forward the entire time. After 3-4 rounds of breath, switch to the other side.

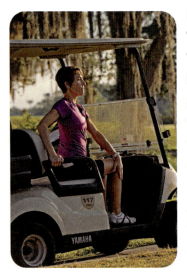

Seated Twist

Twists create space between each vertebra of the spine. They also bring fresh blood flow to many organs and improve digestion. Done in this seated position, you can get all the increased energy and range of motion benefits you would from a standing or floor-based position. Plus, the golf cart provides a perfect seat from which to twist during your round.

Inhale to sit tall. Exhale and take your right hand across your left knee, and your left hand behind you on the chair. Take 5 cycles of breath. Then, inhale to return to center and repeat on the second side.

Down Dog

This Downward-Facing Dog variation is common in many chair yoga classes and is very accessible on the golf course. Stand at the front or back of your cart and place your hands on a level, steady surface. Keep your feet hip distance apart as you walk them further away from the cart. As the torso folds forward, draw the belly button toward your spine to protect your lower back.

The intensity of this stretch is determined by how far you move your feet and hips from the cart. Find a point that elicits a 50-70% stretch and breathe deeply. You will strengthen the arms, core, and hip stabilizing muscles while simultaneously lengthening the sides of the body and hamstrings. You'll need all these actions throughout your round. Then, to come out, slowly walk your feet back toward the cart.

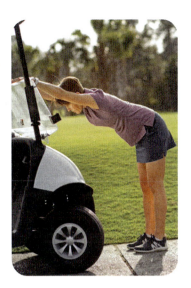

Standing Hip Circles

Stand on a curb next to your cart, holding on to the cart as needed to stay upright.

Make sure your entire left foot is supported by a firm surface beneath you. Then, hover your right foot in space. Your right hip will tend to drop due to gravity. Press your left foot into the ground, draw your left hip toward the midline, and lift your right hip up so it's level with your left. This will return your pelvis to a neutral position.

Now, swing your right leg clockwise in small circles for 5-10 rounds. Keep the rest of your body as stationary as possible. Switch the direction of your circle, moving the right leg counterclockwise for 5-10 rounds. Even though your right leg is moving, your left hip is working to stabilize your entire body. Pause in Mountain Pose before repeating this exercise on the other side. The goal here is small movements that increase awareness in the hips.

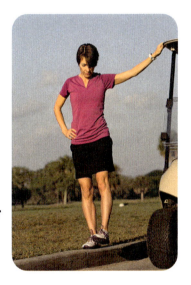

CONSERVE ENERGY ON THE COURSE

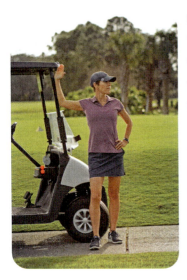

Chest Stretch

The pectoralis muscles commonly get tight because of the golf swing. Use a brief static stretch throughout your round to counteract the forward movement of this muscle group and to improve your posture.

With your right side next to the cart, stand in Mountain Pose and bring your right arm into a Cactus position. Allow your entire forearm to rest against the vertical post of your cart, keeping a 90-degree angle at the shoulder and elbow. Then, inch your entire body forward until you observe sensation at the front of the chest and shoulder. Breathe deeply for 30 seconds. Then repeat on the other side.

Putting it Together

Pause now and take a very deep breath! You just discovered why your focus gets challenged on the golf course. Instead of carrying unwanted baggage like overthinking, distractions, and blame, you can turn your concentration on and off like a light switch to conserve energy. These techniques are simple, yet, they require practice. Point-and-call around your house or breathe on purpose when driving around town. Maybe unroll your yoga mat and try these new yoga postures this week. The goal is to improve your focus long-term, so make sure sure you have fun in the process.

Take Action Now

- **Start with a simple activity.**
  Select one or two methods from the week and practice them at home.

- **Apply your chosen method to golf.**
  As you build confidence with the basics, incorporate one selected method into your next golf game. Observe what mental shifts occur. Take notes in your golf journal or share your experience with a friend. Or, send me an email (Kym@Swagtail.com) with your insights. I love hearing about your progress!

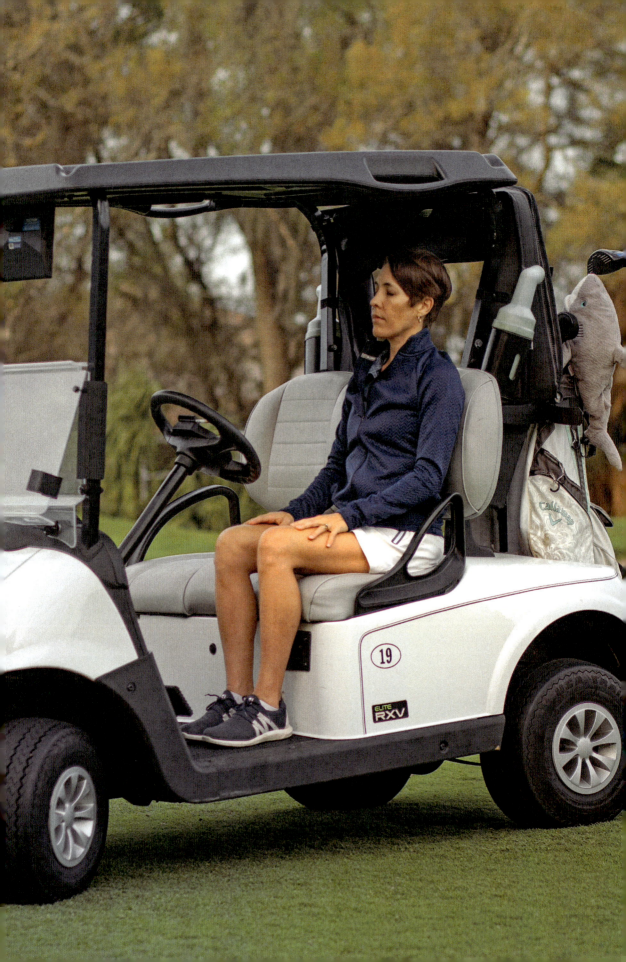

WEEK 5

Post-Round Recovery

"In Western culture, we tend to be consumed by the perspective that the thing we want to happen—getting stronger, faster, fitter—is happening only when we're working on it, exerting some kind of control. We aren't used to the idea that letting go, resting, and relaxing control can be as important to healing, recovery, and strengthening as they are."

—Marvin Zauderer, sports performance coach[1]

WEEK 5 OVERVIEW

Many golfers sink their last putt on hole 18 and consider their rollercoaster of a game complete. Yet, your body and mind need time to adjust from the experience. That's why the tools this week release physical tension, calm the nervous system, and shift your perspective so you can ease into life beyond the course in a balanced, energized way.

Consider this equation: Improvement (training gains) = Stress + Rest.

You just dedicated the past four weeks to learning new yoga-based techniques that challenge your existing patterns. And if you just finished a round of golf, your game was a stress to your system (no matter what your score). Now it's time to rest. Recovery after your round is where your body heals, and you adapt to the new levels of stimuli. This week I'll reveal the exact elements of a post-round recovery ritual that will uplift your body and mind. As a result, you'll have a renewed desire and physical capacity to succeed the next time you hit the golf course. You'll also experience greater health in the interim.

Let me give you a glimpse into my world after a round of golf. Summer is my competitive playing season, and the first thing I do when I get home is jump in the lake. I follow this cold plunge with a warm shower and large glass of water. Then, I plop myself dead center on the living room carpet to stretch.

After ten years of marriage, Steve is familiar with this afternoon routine. He often pours himself a whiskey neat, assumes his position in the recliner behind me, and turns on a Western. Now we can both enjoy the shared space, given our mutual affinity for relaxation and gritty cowboy movies.

Later that evening, I enter my hole-by-hole score into the color-coded Excel spreadsheet on my laptop. Geeky, I know. However, this system allows me to see which holes I'm playing well, and which ones need a new strategy. I then finish the day with a few notes in my journal before bed.

Each of these actions are deliberate in nature. As we go through the elements of a post-round recovery ritual, you'll understand their significance. And given this new information, you'll be able to tailor a post-golf plan that works for you.

The Power of Endings

Many golfers believe that how they start out matters most. Only, endings have incredible power, too. How you end an experience influences what you do and how you do it. As Daniel H. Pink describes in his book, *When*,[2] endings shape your behaviors in four predictable ways.

Endings:

- **Energize:** When endings are near, it's human desire to finish strong. You might have noticed a burst of energy on the last few holes of your round. The goal is to keep that positive momentum going into your post-round ritual, which will set you up to play your best moving forward.
- **Encode:** At the end of any event, it's natural to evaluate what just happened and record important details. We do this on purpose after golf. This way, you view your entire game, including the rough patches, in a positive light. Plus, you generate good-feeling body chemicals that linger long after your round ends.
- **Edit:** Endings edit your experience. It's like cleaning out your golf bag; you keep what matters most and discard the rest so that you start fresh next game. We'll do this with the mind and body in this post-round recovery period.
- **Elevate:** Golf is full of exhilarating and deflating moments alike. You can crumble and miss a two-foot putt one minute, then hit your best drive the next. This blend of emotions keeps you hooked on the game. More importantly, they provide unexpected insights and moments of transcendence that elevate your spirit.

My goal for you is to end each round feeling even better than when you began. The techniques this week will help you do just!

The Recovery Phase

Before exploring those tools, I want you to understand how recovery fits into the big picture of your golf game. Remember, yoga is not your sport. It's a resource you utilize to enhance your golf game. This means you'll want to know *when* and *how* to use yoga-based methods after your round for maximum impact.

Let's say you just completed a round of golf. You have increased the intensity of your body's actions from a baseline norm. Your muscles utilized nutrients to perform your swing, and a whole host of other internal chemical changes took place to sustain your pace of play. As a result, your body has undergone a stressful encounter. It's now time to rebuild your muscles and restore the nervous system through rest.

This recovery period is where this happens. It's when the body repairs muscle fibers, synthesizes proteins and glycogen, and restores hormone levels. Basically, you regain your energy and restore homeostasis in this recovery period. To better understand the timeline of this restoration, look at the four cycles of adaptation.

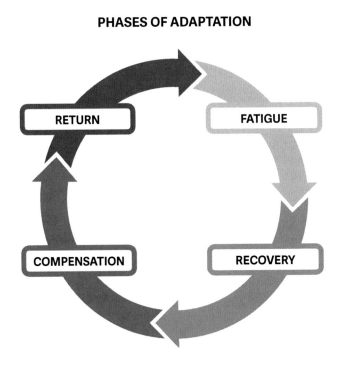

Fatigue (0-2 hrs. after the event)

In this stage, you're tired. Neural activation is reduced and your muscle glycogen reserves are depleted. You also experience mental fatigue, since so much energy was used to focus during your game. In this time frame, your sympathetic nervous system still dominates, and cortisol, the hormone released in conjunction with the stress response, is still high (even if you had a good game).

When you're in fatigue, passive, static stretching can help remove inflammation or swelling caused by the golf swing. Pranayama (breathing techniques) and meditation are a great way to downregulate the nervous system, too.

Recovery (1-2 days after)
The recovery phase is the 24- to 48-hour period that follows your round of golf or intense training. The body continues to use more energy during this period to restore protein and hormonal balance, as well as replenish your energy storehouse. That's why you still want to keep the movements gentle in nature during this time period. The recovery yoga class on page 123 is a great way for the body to recover within the first 48-hours after your round.

Compensation (36-72 hours)
In this time frame, your body has likely adapted physically and mentally to your new level of fitness. Because you feel stronger, greater training levels can be applied. This could be a more intense yoga class, like the cross-training one on page 152. You might even get back on the course for another round of golf, have a lesson with your coach, or return to the range for more specific practice.

Return (3-7 days)
This fourth phase is vital for improvement in golf performance over time. If more training is not applied during this phase, then you lose any previous gains. I suggest you continue with more cross-training yoga classes in this return period. Often this is when you can experience the most growth out on the golf course again.

    The post-round recovery ritual you create this week will be used within 48-hours of your golf game or golf-specific training session.
    Then in week 6, we'll look at ways to balance the intensity of your game with periods of relaxation to help you improve at a maximum rate.

Elements of a Post-Round Recovery Ritual

Recovery after golf is all about returning you to a completely refreshed state. You know, the kind of days where you have a spring in your step and authentic zest behind your actions. The elements of a post-round recovery ritual will help you get there. Ideally, you'll use each within the first 48-hours after your round to get the most benefit.

I use the acronym REST to remember these elements:
- R = Resilience
- E = Equanimity
- S = Self-study
- T = Time-saving practices

When you create a post-round recovery ritual around REST, you're creating a pathway to healing. This is the exact opposite of adding another set of to-do items to your checklist. That's why I recommend you keep your ritual simple. You want it to meet your needs while fitting nicely into your other life events. Ideally, your recovery process will help you save time and give you more energy in the process.

One of the main ways it does this is by shifting your nervous system.

On the golf course, your mind and body encounter stressors. Even on weekly play days at your club or a round with your best friends, your sympathetic nervous system often gets activated.

What's the sympathetic nervous system?

It's your body's fight-or-flight response that puts you on high alert. This system mobilizes your internal resources for action. Your senses heighten and your awareness increases during play. All these natural responses can serve you well to meet—and exceed—the challenges of your game.

While those benefits serve you on the course, living in a sympathetic dominant state leads to chronic stress. Chronic stress then manifests in the body as muscle tension, pain, physical weakness, adrenal fatigue, and reduced immune function.

Chronic stress also affects the mind. It reduces your ability to concentrate and can make you anxious. It can even make you lose sleep. These combined symptoms then negatively impact your relationships, job performance, and athletic prowess on the golf course.

That's why yoga is so important. It shifts your state of being from the sympathetic nervous system dominance to the parasympathetic nervous system dominance. This is known as downregulation. Your heart rate slows, your blood pressure lowers, and your cortisol levels return to normal.

Operating from the parasympathetic state also enhances the body's recovery process, meaning you can prevent unwanted injuries and increase your performance the next time you play. Let's take a look at how each of the four REST elements of your post-round recovery ritual will bring your body back into balance.

THE NERVOUS SYSTEM

	Parasympathetic Nervous System (Relaxed State)	Sympathetic Nervous System (Stress Response)	Ongoing Sympathetic Nervous System Dominance (Chronic Stress)
Brain	Calm mind and efficient neural connections	Initiates "fight or flight" response	Headaches, memory loss, irritability, anxiety
Eyes	Pupils relax and increased perception	Pupils dialate and perception narrows	Fatigue, difficulty sleeping
Heart	Lower heartrate	Increased heart rate	Cardiovascular disease and increased risk of heart attack
Blood Pressure	Decreases	Increases	Artery damage
Airways	Constrict and slow, rhythmic breathing possible	Expand to escape perceieved danger	Rapid, shallow breathing
Liver	Increased bile production to remove waste, and more energy storage	Increased glucose production and release for immediate energy boost	Insulin resistance and increased risk of diabetes
Digestive System	Increased blood flow and improved digestion	Decreased blood flow and less activity	Gas, bloating, nausea, upset stomach, sugar cravings
Reproductive System	Increased blood flow and libido	Decreased blood flow	Loss of sexual desire, infertility
Hormones	Acetylcholine released to slow heart rate	Cortisol released to increase heart rate	Fatigue, weakened immune system, mood imbalances

R = Resilience in the Body

Resilience is the capability for your muscles to spring back into shape. Your muscles have a natural resting length, as you discovered in week 1. Then, when you exert physical energy, such as taking your golf swing over and over again during a round, those working muscles contract (or get shorter) in order to give you power.

A muscle is said to be elastic when it can return to that same resting length quickly after being used.

Many times, though, chronic tension builds in the body and those same muscles cannot return to that normal resting length, which means you get less power over time.

That's why we use yoga in the recovery period after your round to restore the resting length of your muscular tissue.

The types of yoga that are best suited for this recovery period include:

Gentle Yoga. Gentle Yoga consists of slow, deliberate movements to increase circulation after playing. The poses used here also reduce the buildup of lactic acid in the muscles, minimizes post-golf stiffness, and alleviates the fatigue that immediately follows play. Plus, repeating these less-intense poses can counteract inflammation and helps stimulate the immune response to keep you healthy and strong.

Yin Yoga. Yin Yoga works on the deeper tissues of the body, including the ligaments, tendons, and fascia. These tissues can be less elastic and hydrated than muscle. Therefore, poses are taken with less intensity and for longer periods of time to ensure proper stimulation.

Restorative Yoga. This is a relaxing, supportive practice that reprograms the nervous system. This is done by gently stimulating different organs and portions of the body with a light stretch. Numerous props are also used to assist this process, which means that minimal effort is necessary to restore the body's natural capacity for health.

On the surface, Restorative Yoga appears similar to a Yin-style practice. Both hold postures for a more extended period at a fraction of your total capacity. While the body physically opens as a result of these held poses, the goal of Restorative Yoga is not to lengthen the tissues. Instead, it's to help regulate the nervous system.

Quiz: Test Your Fascia Knowledge

It's not just your muscles that adapt to the hours of asymmetrical movements on the golf course. Your repetitive swing can also create an imbalance in your fascia, too. For many years, fascia was viewed as unimportant and thrown away when dissecting cadavers.

But, oh, how the tides have turned. We now understand that fascia is a web-like network that provides balance and structure to your entire body.[3] Your fascia is also highly adaptable. It constantly adjusts so you can remain safe in the face of various physical demands.

The quiz below will test your fascia knowledge. It will also reveal why keeping it healthy is beneficial to your golf game.

Quiz Instructions:

Read each statement below and decide if it is true or false. Once you've marked all 10 statements, compare your answers with the key on the following page (no peeking).

#	Statement	T	F
1	Fascia is the connective tissue of the body.	T	F
2	Fascia is the largest sensory organ in the body.	T	F
3	The purpose of your fascia is to give the body structure, support your organs, and help the body adapt to changing demands in life.	T	F
4	Fascial tissue changes quickly.	T	F
5	Your hydration levels affect the health of your fascia.	T	F
6	Fascia helps regulate immune function in your body.	T	F
7	Cross-links in the fascia are where adjacent tissues become stuck to one another.	T	F
8	Myofascial release (MFR) is a technique designed to remove obstacles in the fascia, increase the flow of nerve signals in the tissue, and restore its overall integrity.	T	F
9	Aggressive, persistent myofascial release can benefit the fascia.	T	F
10	Repetitive movements in yoga can increase fascia health.	T	F

Fascia Answer Key

1. TRUE
Fascia is the connective tissue of the body. A superficial layer runs from head to toe, just under the skin, which protects the body and provides a sense of support. Then, there is a deeper layer that surrounds—and weaves through—all the muscles of the body.

2. TRUE
The body's fascia houses sensory nerves that constantly absorb information from your environment via your senses. In fact, it takes in more data than your brain about the conditions inside of your body AND outside of it! The fascia picks up each small change in your weight, body position, and various movements. It also stores this information to help you sustain homeostasis.

3. TRUE
Your fascia works wonders to keep you alive and well each day. First, it provides a sense of support for the structure of your body. Fascia essentially provides the framework in which your bones, muscles, nerves, and organs connect. Second, it's a layer that surrounds and protects your vital internal organs. This entire network of support allows your body to absorb physical stress without distorting your shape.

4. FALSE
Your fascia is constantly—but slowly—responding to the demands placed on your body. The collagen networks of the fascia rearrange over time to help you move in ways your lifestyle requires. If you're a new mom carrying a baby around for months on end, your fascia will adjust to help your body sustain that load. Or, as a golfer, you must build strength and coordination to perform the intense golf swing. Your fascia adjusts to help you repeat these activities (and more).

5. TRUE
60% of the adult human body is composed of water and staying hydrated can increase your overall health. This is also true for your connective tissue. One component of fascia is collagen fibers, which resist the deformation of the tissue and help your body heal. For collagen to remain healthy, though, you must be hydrated.

Water also comprises a majority of the ground substance found in the fascia. This thick, gel-like fluid fills the space between fibers and cells in this connective tissue and helps the muscles of your body glide past one another smoothly. If you're dehydrated, your muscles will be like sandpaper rubbing against one another (which sounds miserable, right?) Instead, stay hydrated to maintain smooth, coordinated, and efficient body movement.

6. TRUE
White blood cells and fibroblasts are the two main types of cells in the fascia. White blood cells regulate immune function and inflammation in the body. In the deep fascia, myofibroblasts also assist in wound healing. Therefore, healthy fascia can significantly contribute to the immune function of the body. It allows your body to be more resilient in the face of toxins, stress, and damage to tissue from trauma, injury, or simple wear and tear from everyday life activities.

7. TRUE
If you were to look through a microscope at healthy fascia tissue, you'd see packed collagen fibers that form a wavy pattern. This allows the tissue of the fascia—and other tissues of the body, such as muscles—to stretch and move without restriction.

Yet, if cross-links form in the fascia, that healthy movement isn't possible. Crosslinks are adhesions in the tissue and where fascia gets stuck. They act like Velcro in the body and cause tension, pain, and reduced blood flow to the fascial network. Cross-links can occur because of physical trauma, emotional stress, aging, or overuse. To prevent this or heal from injury, you can use myofascial release techniques to repair this tissue.

8. TRUE
Myofascial release (MFR) is any technique you can use to manipulate muscles and fascia. Some MFR techniques include compressing a point on the body with a tennis ball (such as the foot and shoulder exercises in this recovery section) or rolling over a tight muscle with a foam roller.

While there are many ways to use MFR, the main goals are to release adhesions, restore the order of collagen fibers in the tissue, and restore neuromuscular connections. Plus, it's a great way to restore (and increase) the elastic potential of muscles, which translates to more length, strength, and flexibility.

9. FALSE

As you probably know, more isn't always better. This is also true when using MFR techniques to improve fascial health. Try to vary how you address your connective tissue. Sometimes work on a more superficial level. Other times work more deeply. One day you might build strength, the next, mobility.

In any case, you want to avoid an aggressive approach to alter your fascia. It can trigger more inflammation in the body, which results in more internal stress and activates the sympathetic nervous system. This inflammation can delay—or even prevent—the desired healing effect you're after. Therefore, when we use the MFR techniques after golf, we start on the gentler side and slowly increase duration and intensity.

10. FALSE

Yes, it's true. Yoga is one of the best ways to stretch and compress the tissues of the body, including the fascia. Yoga is also a wonderful way to increase balance and overall body awareness. Yet, the best way for fascial health and resilience to be attained is through various movements. You want to use slow, mindful movements of your body in new directions to stress different points on the tension system. Thus, repetitive movements in yoga won't necessarily help improve your fascia. This is why we use a variety of movements on the mat to target fascia in a healthy way.

> *"A successful approach to recovery will depend on two traits: patience and faith. You need patience so you can give your body the time it needs to heal itself. And you need to trust that time off, even though it's hard to take, will have a direct, positive effect on your life [and golf game]."*
>
> – Sage Roundtree, author and yoga teacher

Activity: A Post-Round Recovery Practice

The yoga sequence below incorporates Gentle, Yin, and Restorative yoga to increase resilience in the body. You are retraining the fascia and musculature around your bones in these longer-held postures. The MFR techniques will help with this as well. The most important thing is to set yourself up with your props in advance. This way, you can completely relax and be supported in each pose.

I suggest you read through this section first. Then, I'll lead you through this sequence on the mat. Visit theFlexibleGolfer.com/free to access the class when you're ready.

Time: 60-75 minutes. There is a shorter version on page 133.
Props needed for the sequence:
- Two tennis balls or myofascial release balls (I like the RAD rounds)
- Golf ball
- Yoga strap (a belt or scarf will work)
- Bolster (or stack of firm towels)
- Rolled blanket, towel, or yoga mat

1. Foot Release

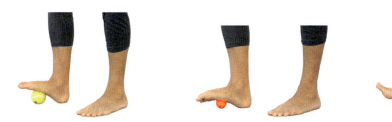

The feet have two critical roles: bearing your body weight and propelling your movement. Unwanted tension—caused by overactivity, injury, or poorly-fitted shoes—can hinder both functions. That's why it's essential to address the fascia in the feet between rounds.

The fascia on the underside of the feet continues up the back of the calves, hamstrings, sacrum, and entire back line of the body. Thus, when you release tension in the feet, you positively affect these other areas as well.

Start with a golf ball or tennis ball:
- Stand or sit with both feet on the ground. Notice any sensations on the underside of each foot.

- Place the ball under the center of one foot. Lean into the ball to increase the pressure. Ease your weight on that foot to make it easier. You can curl or extend your toes to modify the sensations, as well. Find any tender area and stay for 30-60 seconds.
- Gently roll the ball under as much surface area on the bottom of that foot as possible. Continue this technique for about 1 minute.
- Remove the ball from under your foot. Stand or sit in your starting position. Observe any new sensations in the feet or legs.
- Repeat the same movements with the other foot.

2. Staff Pose

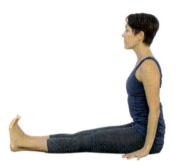

Also known as Dandasana, Staff Pose is a symmetrical way to set the tone for the upcoming seated postures. It also lengthens the spine and hamstrings while encouraging good posture.

Start seated on your mat:
- Extend your legs out in front of the torso. Keep them together and lightly flex the feet. Point your toes up. If your torso is leaning backward, sit on a blanket or bend the knees slightly.
- Anchor both sitting bones and lengthen the spine. Broaden the collarbones. Palms press lightly into the floor.
- Without harboring tension, breathe here for 1 minute.

3. Seated Twist

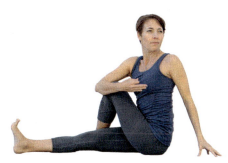

You just spent hours on the golf course actively twisting the spine for your swing. Now it's time to relax into one. Doing so in this variation will stretch the back, outer hips, glutes, and hamstrings (all of which worked on the course to help you swing).

Start in Staff Pose:
- Take your right foot and cross it over your left thigh so that the entire foot can rest on the ground. Keep both sitting bones grounded and your spine long
- Use your exhale to twist to your right. Your left elbow can hook around your bent right knee for support, and your right hand can rest gently on the floor outside your right hip. Ideally, use your core strength to keep the pelvis neutral (not rocking back).
- Hold the pose for 2-3 minutes. Then move to pose 4. I promise we'll repeat the other side in just a few minutes.

4. Half Cow Face Pose Variation

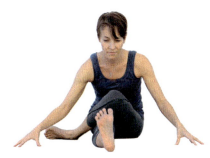

Ready to go deeper still into a low back release and outer hip stretch? Want more length in the hamstrings? This pose will give you all of this, plus room to calm the mind since the pose is a forward fold.

Keep your left leg extended and drop your right knee over your left (as close as it can get comfortably). Your right foot will likely end up somewhere outside of your left hip. Your spine will remain tall at first with your sitting bones pressing down into the mat. Then, fold forward to any degree where you feel a gentle stretch at the back of your left leg, outer right hip, or low back. The tightest area of your body will give you feedback first. Continue to breathe deeply here for 2-3 minutes.

5. Repeat Poses 3 and 4 on the Other Side

You've twisted to the right and taken a fold with the right leg on top. Now, it's time to even out your body. First, set yourself up to twist to the left. Then, after holding the seated twist for the same amount of time you took on the right, lower the left knee over the extended right leg and fold.

6. Seated Forward Fold

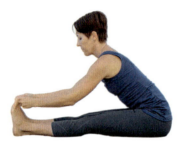

This yoga pose lengthens the entire back line of the body symmetrically. It further releases any hamstring, low back, upper back, and neck tension that might have accumulated during your game.

Begin in Staff Pose:
- Anchor the sitting bones and back of the legs into the floor. Keep the spine long, and the chest open as you start to hinge the pelvis forward. Lengthen the front of the body as you continue to fold. Just make sure you can sustain a calm, deep rhythm of breath wherever you are. Bending the knees or sitting on a blanket can make this easier.
- Stay in the pose for 1-3 minutes.

7. Rhomboid Release

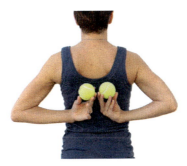

The rhomboid muscles between the shoulder blades provide mobility and stability when you swing your golf club. This area can harbor tension as a result. The rhomboid release is also a great activity to offset hours in a seated position or improve overall posture.

Start with two tennis balls:
- Lie on your back, with your knees bent and the soles of your feet on the ground. Lift your hips and place the tennis balls on either side of the spine, just below the level of the shoulder blades.
- Relax completely. Let the weight of your body intensify the sensations.
- If you are happy there, you can slowly begin making large circles with the arms. Just make sure you can breathe deeply and remain relaxed.
- You can then shift the hips down on your mat so that the tennis balls are now 2-3 inches higher than they were previously. Rest and breathe here. Arm circles are also an option in this new position to further release tension.

8. Rotator Cuff Release

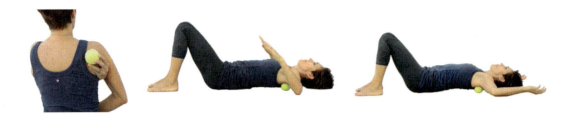

The rotator cuff muscles are the smaller group that keeps your shoulder girdle steady and mobile at the same time. The exercise here specifically releases the infraspinatus and teres minor that often get strained in shoulder injuries (see page 36). Better still, practice these movements often to prevent injury in the first place.

Use two tennis balls:
- Lie on your back, knees bent, and feet on the floor.
- Place each tennis ball behind the meaty portion of your shoulder blade, just below the horizontal bone you can feel with your hand. Again, relax your muscles and allow your body weight to apply pressure on the tennis balls. Slowly roll around until you find a tender area. Then stay and breathe.
- Once you can relax into those sensations, bring your arms out to the side in a bent, cactus-shaped position. If comfortable, bring the hands overhead. Next, move the forearms and hands to point forward your feet, all the while keeping your elbows on the ground. Repeat 5-10 times.
- Remove the tennis balls and breathe deeply for about 1 minute. Notice any sensations around the shoulder region.

9. Reclined Hamstring Stretch

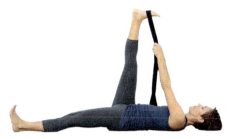

Also known as the Reclined Hand-to-Big-Toe Pose, this posture relieves compression and tension in the low back. It also opens the hamstrings on the lifted leg and can lengthen the quadriceps on the lower leg (if kept straight).

Lie on your back:
- Bend your knees and place the soles of both feet on the floor.
- Hug your right knee into your chest and place your yoga strap around the ball of your foot.
- Extend your right leg toward the ceiling, straightening it only as much as 50-70% of your capacity. Your left knee can remain bent. Or, straighten the left leg along the floor to intensify the stretch.
- Stay for 3-5 minutes on the right side before switching to the left.

10. Restorative Side-Lying Stretch

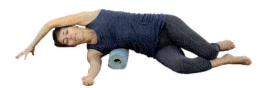

This side-lying stretch releases any tension in the intercostal muscles to make breathing easier.

Grab your bolster or a rolled yoga mat:
- Place the bolster or rolled yoga mat underneath your side ribs, with its long edge parallel to your spine. Have your block or blanket nearby, as well.
- With your hips on the floor and knees comfortably bent, rest your side ribs on the bolster. Adjust the position of the block/blanket so your head can rest on it.
- Let your bottom shoulder hang toward the floor.

- Allow the top arm to rest on your side, or if comfortable for the shoulder, raise it overhead so that it can rest on the floor or a prop.
- Stay and breathe deeply for 3-5 minutes.
- Move to the other side when you're ready and stay for the same length of time.

11. Reclined Butterfly Pose

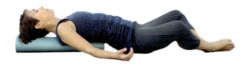

In Yin Yoga, this pose is known as Reclined Butterfly Pose. It's yet another way to open the chest after the rounding that often occurs when you swing a golf club. The abdomen and pelvis relax. Plus, the inner groin muscles re-lengthen after the engagement used to stabilize your stance when swinging.

Use a rolled blanket or yoga mat:
- Place your support in a vertical position behind the spine. Ideally, the back of the head and ribcage will be supported by it, and the low back can hang freely to release any tension in this area. The back of the pelvis will rest on the ground.
- Bend the knees and place the soles of the feet together. Arms can rest out to the sides, straight or bent.
- You can place a blanket under the back of your head for more comfort. You can also set blocks behind the knees for additional support.

12. Reclined Figure-4 Pose

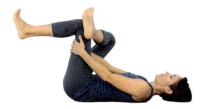

The hip stabilizers worked hard during your golf game to keep your swing steady. Now it's time to elongate this muscle group. In particular, the piriformis lengthens and the sciatic nerve does, too. The lower back also releases in this supine position.

Begin on your back with your feet on the floor:
- Cross your lower right leg, just above the ankle, on your left quadriceps. Keep the right foot flexed. Stay here if you already notice a deep stretch in the outer right hip.
- To move on, draw the left knee toward your chest, reach between the inner thighs and grab anywhere behind the left hamstrings. Keep moving the right knee out to the side while keeping the back of the pelvis evenly on the ground.
- Stay for 2-4 minutes on this side. Then repeat with the left leg over right.

13. Reclined Twist

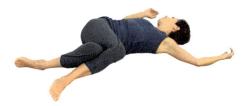

Not only does this Reclined Twist further stretch the gluteus maximus, but it also elongates the sides of the abdomen, pectoral muscles, and neck.

Start in constructive rest, on your back with the feet flat on the floor.
- Lift your hips and shift them two inches to the right. Then, drop your knees over to the left. A block or blanket can be placed under the knees, or between them, for more support.
- Extend the arms out to your sides and allow gravity to drop the back of your shoulders toward the ground. Let your head rest completely. Stay for 2-5 minutes on the first side, then switch.

14. Legs Up The Wall Pose

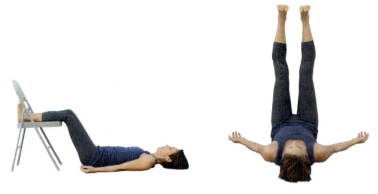

This is one of the best poses to revive the lower body after a long day on the golf course. You get upside down, which shifts your perspective, and the flow of circulation effortlessly brings blood back to the heart. Your nervous system also calms down into a restful state.

First, decide if you will put your legs up the wall or on a chair.

Then, sit with your side of the body next to the wall or chair and begin to recline down onto your back. Due to the lack of space, you will be forced to swing your legs up the wall or place them on to the seat of the chair. Allow the low back, pelvis, and legs to relax as much as possible. Your arms can remain in any position that's comfortable to you. Breathe deeply for 4-8 minutes as you let all tension from your game melt away.

15. Final Relaxation

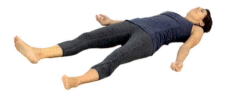

Savasana, or Corpse Pose, might be the easiest yoga posture for the body, yet the most challenging for the mind. In this final relaxation, you want to rest every muscle. You want gravity to pull your body downward, And, you want your breathing to be effortless.

Then, as you're supported by the ground beneath you, focus on your breathing. This is when you absorb the physiological changes of your recovery-based yoga practice. Basically, your body memorizes the new settings you established on the mat, and gives you a new operating system moving forward that is more efficient, powerful, and aligned.

Lie comfortably on your back.

Notice your heels, calves, thighs, buttocks, thoracic spine, shoulder blades, and back of the skull get heavier. Notice which part of your arms touch the ground as the palms face up.

Make yourself as symmetrical as possible. Then, continue to breathe naturally for 3-10 minutes as you rest.

Shorter Recovery Yoga Sequence

Want to recover after your round but don't have a full hour to do so? Shorten the sequence above into a 25-30 minute yoga session.

1. Foot Release (2 minutes each foot)
2. Reclined Hamstring Stretch (1-3 minutes each side)
3. Restorative Side-Lying Sequence (1-3 minutes each side)
4. Reclined Butterfly (3 minutes)
5. Reclined Figure-4 Pose (2-3 minutes each side)
6. Reclined Twist (2-3 minutes each side)
7. Final Relaxation (3 minutes)

More Ways to Increase Resilience in the Body

Yoga is just one of the many ways to help the body and mind recover after your round. Here are some other self-care practices you can do as well:

- Drink more water. Hydration is critical to your performance and recovery.
- Eat a nutritious meal. Ideally, you want to eat a recovery snack within 2 hours of your round—one that is a mixture of carbohydrates, some protein, and minimal fat.
- Ice your muscles or soak in cold water. Cold counters inflammation and numbs pain. Ice for 10-15 minutes at a time, up to three times per day, and lay a thin towel between the ice and your skin to prevent frostbite.
- Take a hot bath or shower. Heat can relax muscles and the mind while boosting circulation. However, applying heat to already inflamed areas can slow recovery time.
- Get a massage. Deliberate bodywork can reduce adhesions and muscle cramping. This is a great supplement to your overall health, as your budget and schedule allow.

E = Equanimity of the Mind

The second component of your recovery ritual involves resting the mind. Equanimity is about being calm and composed under all circumstances, including challenging ones. Our goal is to return to this state and release any mental stress that accumulated during your round. We'll do this through breathwork.

Activity: Breathing to Calm the Mind

Last week, we used an even, deliberate breathing pattern to remain composed on the course. Now we're going to change this rhythm. In this activity, the exhale will become longer than the inhale. This induces the relaxation response and calms the mind.

Time Frame: 5-15 minutes

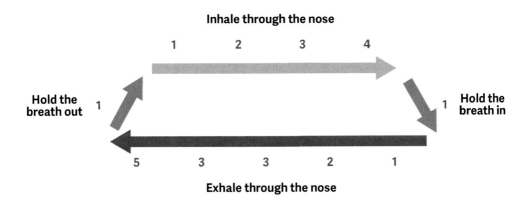

Step 1: Establish Your Position
Find a comfortable, seated position. Keep your spine tall and broaden your collarbones. Then let your hands rest effortlessly in your lap.

Step 2: Observe Your Baseline Breathing
Notice the natural rhythm of your breath. Without changing that rhythm in any way, notice how long it takes you to breathe in. Observe how long it takes to breathe out.

Step 3: Elongate the Exhale
Count how long it takes you to breathe in naturally. Then, pause for a count of 1 while you hold the breath in. Then slow down the exhale, so it becomes longer than your inhale. If you inhaled to a count of 2, exhale to a count of 3. If you inhaled to a count of 4, exhale to a count of 5. You can start with a single count longer on your exhale. Maybe you can extend that outbreath two counts longer than the inhale. Be sure no strain results from your breathing, though. Then, pause for a count of 1 before you breathe in again.

Repeat your breathing pattern for 1-2 minutes.

Step 4: Observe the Effects

As you return to your natural, effortless pace of breathing, notice any new sensations in the body. Become aware of your new state of mind. The shifts might be subtle at first. Yet, with practice, the effects of deliberate breathing can lead to dramatic improvements in your overall well-being.

You can return to this breathing exercise anytime you want to reduce mental stress. I also suggest you pair it with the recovery yoga sequence this week. For example, you can take a few rounds of a slower exhale before you start the practice. Or, you can incorporate it before Savasana (Corpse Pose) to deepen the relaxation response at the end of your recovery class.

S = Self-Study

The next element of your post-round recovery ritual is self-study. In traditional yogic texts, this practice is known as Svadyaya. Reflection is so essential in yoga that it's included in one of the eight limbs of the practice (see page 16).

Self-study is where you use your conscious mind to review your round, allowing you to synthesize what you learned on the course. It also gives you greater awareness of where to bolster your game moving forward. By now, you know that attention is a critical component for success in both yoga and golf. Reflection refines your focus, and it's a technique that helps you stay the course toward mastery.

Many times, the very moment you feel like you have mastered a skill in golf is the very same instant you're likely to become complacent about it. This is why it's essential to reflect on your progress.

You want to review your habits and make adjustments continually to play the absolute best you can in your golf game.

After your game, use a journal or blank sheet of paper to answer the following questions:

- What were my three best shots today?
- Which sensations in my body are most noticeable now?
- Did I manage my energy levels well on the course? Why or why not?
- When was I most focused during my round?

One of my favorite quotes is by Søren Kierkegaard, which says, *"Life can only be understood backwards, but it must be lived forwards."*[4] This means you can use self-study to gain knowledge about yourself as a golfer. However, it's what you do with that information that matters.

Take the insights from your answers above and pick one thing you can do now to improve your performance. It could be to get on your mat and stretch the body to ease any pain. You share your best shots with a loved one, and explain why those shots went so well for you (Hint: verbalizing your great moments further engrains them in the subconscious mind for later use). You might even adjust your pre-round routine to ensure you're more prepared next round. Just be sure you remain playful as you learn and grow!

T = Time-Saving Practices

The last of the four elements of your post-round recovery ritual is logistical. These time-saving tips help you remain organized as a golfer and prepare you, in advance, for your next round.

This reminds me of the many years I packed my lunch for school. Instead of waking up early in the morning to do this, my mom encouraged me to pack my lunch the night before. I would get out the bread, peanut butter, and jelly. I'd grab an apple, string cheese stick, and a chewy chocolate chip cookie from mom's fresh made batch. Then, each item was carefully arranged in my bright pink Hello Kitty lunchbox and placed in the refrigerator for safekeeping.

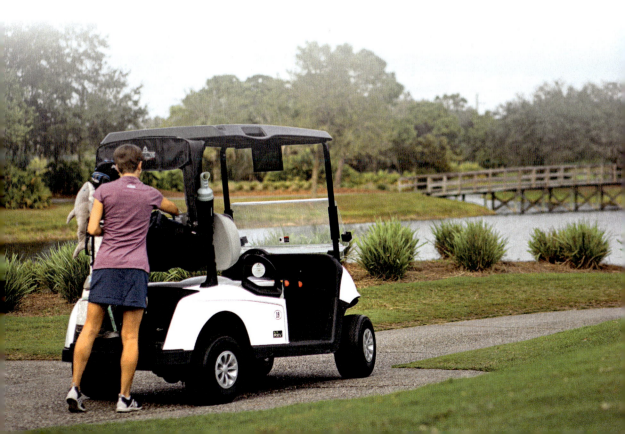

Since my lunch was already packed come morning, I had more time and energy to get ready for the day. Similarly, cleaning up the logistical elements immediately following play saves you mental and physical energy before starting your next round.

You likely take some of these steps already. For example, you drive the cart to your car, have your clubs cleaned by the cart attendant (or do so yourself), unload your clubs, and put everything back in your bag.

Here are some additional logistics you can incorporate after your game to save time when you show up to play next:

Clean Your Clubs

It may seem obvious, but you want to ensure your clubs get cleaned. Make sure your club head covers are also back on the right clubs, and your clubs are in the proper place in your bag.

Empty the Cart

Next, you want to make sure you have emptied the cart, so you don't leave anything valuable at the course. This also includes emptying your pockets—no more orphaned tees in the car, on your nightstand, or kitchen counter.

Replace Your Golf Towel

My third recommendation is to have your golf towel replaced immediately after play. I keep three or four fresh towels in my golf bag at all times. At the end of my game, I remove the dirty towel and reach for a fresh one. This might seem like a small step, but it saves me time when I'm ready to play again.

Change Shoes and Socks

Over the past few weeks, we've given much attention to your feet. The reason is that they pick up sensory input from your environment and affect your body's awareness, balance, and coordination. If you want these benefits on the golf course, it starts with taking care of your feet when off of it.

We do this with the MFR work on page 123. Only, you might not be able to complete those exercises until you get home. That's why I suggest you change your socks and shoes immediately following play. Even let your feet breathe by stepping into a fresh pair of sandals. The goal is to change the sensations at your feet and prevent unwanted bacteria from breeding inside your shoes.

Wash Your Hands and Face

If you're not showering at the clubhouse, I recommend you take the time to wash your hands and face immediately after play. This removes the dirt and sweat that has accumulated during the round. And it will make it much more enjoyable to socialize with friends at the 19th hole if you feel clean. Saucha, or cleanliness, is so important it's also one of the eight limbs of yoga we addressed earlier.

Customize Your Recovery Ritual

Now it's up to you to create your own post-round recovery ritual—one that includes resilience for the body, equanimity of mind, study of the self, and logistical steps to save time. You can use the checklist on the next page to customize these elements in a way that works best with your preferences and lifestyle.

Post-Round Recovery Checklist

Select items that fit within the time frame you have available and are most enjoyable.

R = Resilience of the body (30-90 minutes)

Create resilience in the muscles and fascia after moving asymmetrically in golf.
- ☐ A recovery-focused yoga practice (chair- or floor-based)
- ☐ Drink water
- ☐ Eat a nutritious meal
- ☐ Take a hot bath, shower, soak in a hot tub
- ☐ Ice muscles, cold shower, swim in the lake
- ☐ Get a massage
- ☐ Use myofascial release (MFR) techniques

E = Equanimity in the Mind (5-15 minutes)

Calm the mind and downregulate the nervous system.
- ☐ Breathing techniques that elongate the exhale

S = Self-Study, or Svadyaya (5-15 minutes)

Reflection is a way to increase awareness of both your body and the day's golf experience.
- ☐ What were my three best shots of the game?
- ☐ When was I the most focused during the round?
- ☐ Did I manage my energy levels well on the course? Why/why not?

T = Time-Saving Activities (5- 20 minutes)

Organize your bag and gear so you can start your next round with greater ease.
- ☐ Clean clubs
- ☐ Empty pockets and cart, and ensure all items are returned to the proper place
- ☐ Remove the dirty towel on your bag and replace with a clean one
- ☐ Change socks and shoes
- ☐ Wash hands (and face)

Putting it Together

The recovery period is the important time after your round to recuperate. This is the time for you to REST. It's when your body can release the stress that accumulated during your game. It's also a way for the mind to restore equanimity, reflect on the past with a neutral gaze, and prepare for the future with clarity.

> ## Take Action Now
>
> ❑ **Create a plan for yourself first.**
> Use the provided checklist to create a post-round recovery ritual that matches the time and resources available to you. Keep in mind that you might need to stock up on supplies for your recovery ritual. This could mean gathering additional yoga props or packing snacks in advance. Be sure to have fun with this and be realistic at the same time. Small, simple steps can have a huge impact on future performance.
>
> ❑ **Set time aside on your calendar to recover.**
> Block off time immediately after your round, or within 48-hours of play, to do so. Then give your recovery ritual a try after your next game.

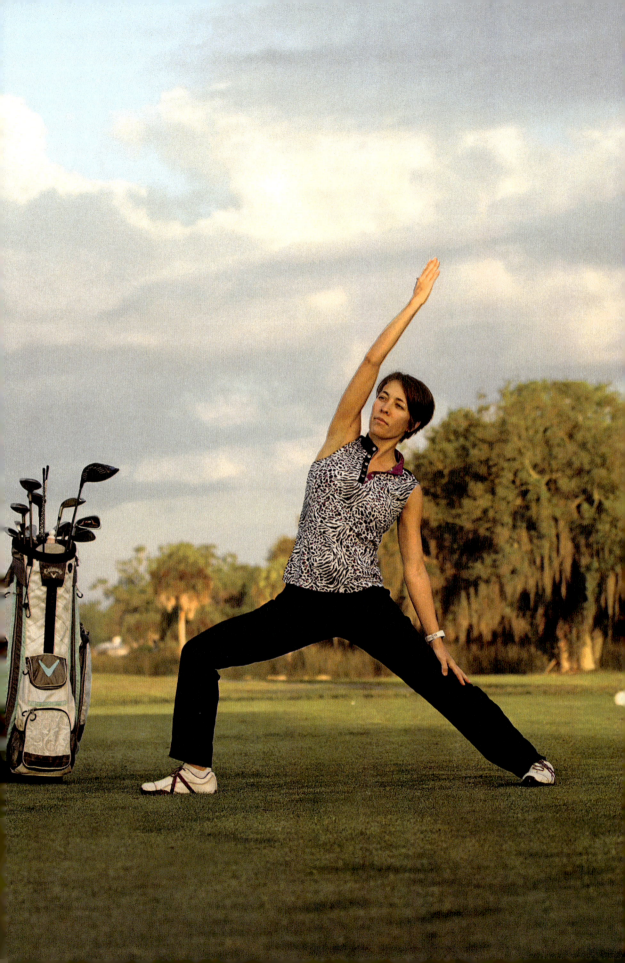

WEEK 6

Stay Golf-Ready All Year Long

"Practice time is when you put your brain into your muscles."

–Sam Snead, professional golfer[1]

WEEK 6 OVERVIEW

Many golfers don't think twice about their next round until they set another tee time, or worse, when they physically return to the course. Yet, your actions between rounds significantly impact future play. That's why this week we'll create a yoga cross-training plan that balances the body, sharpens the mind, and keeps you golf-ready all year long.

Before we dive into cross-training this week—what it is and how you can use it to support your game—I want to take you back to my pre-golf days. Imagine me as a scrawny 6th grader with long blonde hair and a toothy smile. At the wise age of 11, I was ready to trade in my community soccer jersey for one of a competitive team. All I had to do was show my skills in tryouts.

The details of the actual event are a blur in my memory bank. However, I made the team and dedicated the next seven years of my life to the Palos Verdes Breakers. Soccer was my whole life. We played year-round, and in our short off-season, I joined the cross-country team for their running workouts. My short breaks involved eating a pint of Ben and Jerry's cookie dough ice cream on Saturday nights with my best friend, Courtney.

The short story: by high school graduation, I was burned out.

I was well-coached on how to push hard and maximize performance. However, stretching, stress-management, and recovery were overlooked. It wasn't until I found yoga in college that the balance between action and rest really took hold.

Yoga gave me a plan to stay focused.

I like plans because they help you stay on track. They provide structure and purpose. They also save time and energy.

Together, we established a few of these plans over the past few weeks. You created a system to start each round on purpose. This is your pre-round routine. You crafted a path to recovery with your post-round ritual. Now we'll construct a cross-training plan to promote optimal health between rounds.

YOGA CROSS-TRAINING

Cross-training refers to a broad range of activities that increase your fitness. It's an exercise plan designed to move your body in various ways to improve your health. Most importantly, cross-training is a tool that enhances your ability to play well on the course.

This is relevant because you swing your club in one direction for hours on end, creating imbalance. A cross-training routine steps in to support the motions you take on the course—building strength and mobility where needed. It also incorporates actions that complement these movements. This makes you more well-rounded as an individual and helps you avoid injuries.

Cross-training is different from CrossFit. I won't suggest you roll tractor tires through your neighborhood or practice rope climbs in the backyard. Although, if that style of training calls your name, go with your intuition.

I'm here to tell you that not all cross-training is high intensity. I also want to show you how yoga can be one of the best activities to utilize between rounds to support your golf game. We just want to be deliberate about how we use it. You want to know which yoga styles and intensity levels to use, and when to use them.

Said another way, a yoga cross-training plan involves three elements:
- Frequency (how often you practice)
- Intensity (how hard you practice)
- Duration (how long each yoga session lasts)

How you utilize each of these elements depends on the goals you have for yourself as a golfer.

We'll get to that in a minute. First, I want you to understand where yoga cross-training best fits into your week, which is true regardless of your unique goals.

Balance Between Work and Rest

Remember the phases of adaptation we discussed last week? The diagram on page 114 refers to the cyclical patterns of our energy. Cycles are nothing new. All of life moves in a cyclical pattern. We witness changes in the daylight every 24-hours and the shifting seasons each year. Our bodies also fluctuate. There are times we play, train, or work. And there are times we rest.

The recovery phase is how we manage stress and adapt to new challenges. We use relaxation techniques to restore the nervous system, build up our energy supply, and prevent burnout. This is why we use gentle yoga within 48-hours of your golf game or training session.

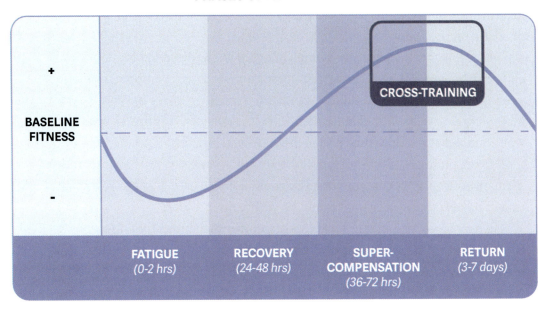

Next, we enter the phases of supercompensation and return where yoga cross-training activities are best applied. Somewhere between 36- to 72-hours after your round, your body has successfully adapted. Your physical stamina is renewed. You're ready to focus mentally and ready to build on your existing skill set.

This window of opportunity overflows into the first portion of the return phase, which lasts 3-7 days after your round. If you don't use yoga cross-training or more specific golf practice in this timeframe, your body will return to its baseline fitness.

That's why we'll create a custom cross-training plan that fits your schedule and physical demands. We won't push too hard, too quickly, and undermine your body's strength. And we won't wait too long, or go too easy, and hinder potential progress. We'll find that sweet spot for your lifestyle so you can recover well, train smart, and maximize your well-being.

Set Your Intention

Before you create a cross-training plan, you want to have a clear intention for yourself as a golfer. If you're here to incorporate yoga into your life to boost general health, start simple. Or, if you're in an extremely busy time period, you might not have the bandwidth to do more. That's completely fine. Research shows that incorporating yoga as little as twice per week can increase your flexibility.[2] Just doing it once each week can sustain any previous gains as well.[3]

If this is the case for you, I suggest you begin with a basic yoga cross-training plan. It could look something like this:

BASIC CROSS-TRAINING PLAN

SUNDAY	MONDAY	TUESDAY	WEDNESDAY	THURSDAY	FRIDAY	SATURDAY
Golf	Recovery yoga 30 min	Off	Off	Yoga cross-training 45 min	Off	Off

If golf is more integrated into your everyday life, or you want to make more distinct changes to your golf-ready body and your golf performance, you can do so with the tools in the next section. In either case, we'll all meet up on the yoga mat for the cross-training class on page 152.

Create a Custom Plan

Golf is an infinite game.[4] You can play year-round, unless your local course is covered in snow, and you can remain a golfer throughout your lifetime. There is no set season of play. There are no finish lines or final buzzers. Without an endpoint, it can be difficult to know how to train.

The good news is that you can formulate a structure for yourself. You decide when to play golf and when to rest. Your cross-training schedule then becomes a support system to help you reach your goals and stay excited to play for many years to come.

There are two cycles that I suggest you create.

Macrocycle

The first is a macrocycle. This is an annual training plan, and it encompasses the twelve-month variations in your game and life. For example, I know that my summer season is when I play golf competitively in my ladies' league. Our course opens at the beginning of May and closes at the end of October. During those six months, I concentrate on refining my skills and improving my score.

CROSS-TRAINING YEARLY SCHEDULE

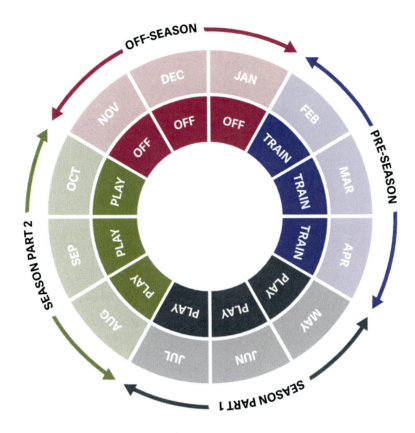

As you know, it's important to treat recovery as part of your training program. This is why I take three months off after my golf season to enjoy other pursuits. I take long bike rides and walks by the beach. I also practice yoga daily. If you live in snow country, you might downhill ski, snowshoe, or join a bowling league in your off-season. The goal is to move the body in a variety of fun ways (and to let your mind focus on something other than golf).

Then, come February, I'm ready to start preparing for my golf season ahead. I ramp up the intensity of my yoga classes and add more cardiovascular exercise, like long walks, to my routine. I also work with my coach to brush off any dust that accumulated from my time off. Since I'm in Florida for some of the winter, I get back out on the golf course at this time. My focus is more skill-based, and my intention is to leisurely explore local courses with my husband as I practice new techniques.

Your annual cycle will likely look very different from mine, and it can change year-to-year. That's okay. The point is to first create broad, distinct phases. So ask yourself:

- What intentions do I have for myself as a golfer in the upcoming year?
- Are there natural shifts in my energy, time frame, and accessibility to golf that could affect my cross-training schedule?
- Is there a season in which I play golf more than others?
- What smaller goals exist within each phase of my year?

With this clarity, you can set a cross-training plan that sustains your energy during each portion of the year.

Microcycle

These smaller cross-training formulas are called microcycles. Over the course of each week, you want to plan challenging and easier activity days. The difficult days target strength and power. They test your body physically and mentally. The light days then give your body time to recover. By creating a schedule for these types of activities, you prevent boredom, burnout, and lower-performance days on the course.

The yoga cross-training sequences this week are moderate workouts. They are designed to squeeze in between your easy and harder activity days and help you retain the elements of a golf-ready body.

Here is a sample of my average week during the off-season. I move in a variety of ways most days of the week. And, because of my age and current fitness level, I tolerate more moderate-to-intense training.

OFF-SEASON WEEKLY SCHEDULE

SUNDAY OFF	MONDAY EASY	TUESDAY MODERATE	WEDNESDAY OFF	THURSDAY MODERATE	FRIDAY MODERATE	SATURDAY EASY
Family day	Recovery yoga 30 min	Yoga cross-training 60 min	Beach day	Light activity 45-60 min	Yoga cross-training 60 min	Recovery yoga 30 min

STAY GOLF-READY ALL YEAR LONG

Next, my pre-season schedule involves more golf-specific training activities. I stick with my yoga cross-training classes, and I add more intensity to them as my energy levels allow.

PRE-SEASON WEEKLY SCHEDULE

SUNDAY OFF	MONDAY HARD	TUESDAY EASY	WEDNESDAY MODERATE	THURSDAY HARD	FRIDAY EASY	SATURDAY MODERATE
Family day	Golf lesson 60 min + Myofascial release 30 min	Yoga recovery class 60-75 min	Cross-training yoga 60-75 min	Golf practice 60 min + Myofascial release 30 min	Yoga recovery class 60-75 min	Cross-training yoga 60-75 min

Then, during my dedicated playing season, time on the practice green, range, and golf course increases dramatically. This means that yoga cross-training takes a back seat. Instead, I focus more on recovery and ways to use yoga to supplement my golf game.

IN-SEASON WEEKLY SCHEDULE

SUNDAY HARD	MONDAY HARD	TUESDAY EASY	WEDNESDAY HARD	THURSDAY EASY	FRIDAY MODERATE	SATURDAY OFF
Golf game 5 hrs + Myofascial release 30 min	Golf game 5 hrs	Yoga recovery class 60 min	Golf lesson 60 min + Myofascial release 30 min	Yoga recovery class 60 min	Easy golf practice 60 min + Yoga cross-training 60 min	Off

Your microcycles could look entirely different. You might spend far more time on the golf course year-round and only weave yoga into your schedule once or twice each week (and for much smaller doses of time). The biggest win comes by creating a plan that works for you—one that honors your age, golf history, present injuries, recovery rate, and overall golf goals.

I also recommend you make at least one week easier than the other three each month. This is especially true during your season of play when you're more active, and it serves as a deeper period of rest for your system. If you don't, your muscles can become tired, tense, and unable to perform. Intentional rest periods prevent that from happening.

Here's a quick review before we move on:
- Recovery yoga classes are perfect for easy days of training or within 48-hours of an intense golf game.
- Moderate yoga cross-training classes are designed to fit between the lighter and harder activity days during the week to sustain, and build, your stamina.

Cross-Training for the Body

Now that you have an idea of how frequently to practice yoga and what intensity to do so, it's time to get on your mat and learn the moves. The cross-training sequence this week is moderate in nature. We'll blend dynamic stretching to warm up the body. Then we'll utilize longer holds to create semi-permanent changes in the tissue. Research demonstrates that you still receive incredible benefits when stretching at 30-40% of your total capacity.[5] In fact, stretching to the point of pain is counterproductive.

Activity: Yoga Cross-Training Sequence

This yoga sequence incorporates a wide array of movements to increase range of motion in the body. We also build strength in the areas needed for your golf swing and release tension in regions that get overworked. If you have physical limitations or difficulty getting up and down from the floor, I recommend starting with the chair yoga sequence on page 163. And if all of this appears overwhelming, that's likely because it's new to you. Take a deep breath and trust that the practice gets easier with repetition.

Time: 60 minutes
Suggested props: Two blocks, a strap

1. Seated Breathing

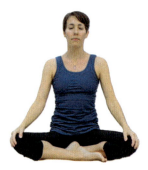

Leave behind the activities and conversations of the past and tune into your breathing. Set an intention for your time on the mat. Thank yourself for carving out this time to improve yourself and your golf game.

Breathe mindfully here for 1-3 minutes. You can simply be aware of your breathing at first. Then start to breathe in and out through the nose. Sustain nostril breathing throughout your cross-training practice.

2. Engage the Core

Recline on to your back. Then use the same toe-tapping technique from page 40 to build heat in your core. Do 8 rounds per side.

3. Reclined Spinal Twist

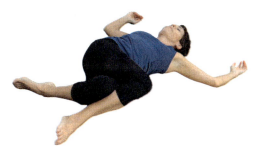

A Reclined Spinal Twist massages the abdominal region you just worked. Plus, it begins to open the hips, side body, and chest while rehydrating the tissue around the spine. Bend both knees together, or cross one leg over the other. Drop the back of the shoulders toward the floor and gaze up or away from your bent knees. Stay for 5-10 breaths on each side.

4. Standing Forward Fold

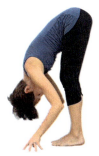

Lengthen the entire back line of the body in this standing Forward Fold. As you spend extra time here, you'll notice where you have tension in the body. Breathe deeply into those areas and envision more spaciousness in the tissue. Let the head hang heavy as you press the floor away with your feet. Remember to bend the knees as much as needed to keep the hips over the feet in space.

5. Half Sun Salute

Increase your circulation and build heat with Half Sun Salutes. See page 75 for details. Repeat 3-5 times.

6. Downward-Facing Dog

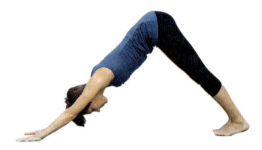

Nicknamed Down-Dog, this pose strengthens the entire body—lats, shoulders, arms, abdomen and legs. Drop your heels toward the ground and bend your knees as much as necessary for the hips to lift. Draw the belly button toward the spine. Keep space between the shoulders and the ears as you push your hands into the mat. Let your head remain heavy, too. Stay for 8 cycles of breath.

7. Child's Pose

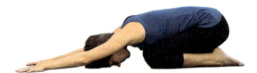

Child's Pose is a resting pose that can be used anytime you need a break in your yoga practice. Your spine lengthens, and you get a gentle compression for the front of the body. You might also sense greater ease with your head supported by the ground (or a block). Just make sure there is no pain in your knees or ankles. Take 10 cycles of breath.

8. Bird Dog

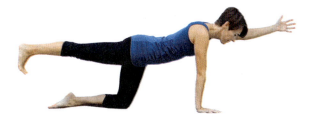

This pose is often referred to as Tabletop Extension. It's an important way to strengthen the low back stabilizing muscles and treat/prevent lower back pain. Bird Dog also creates a strong, functional core that supports you on the golf course.

Lift the opposite leg and arm so that both are parallel to the floor. Draw your belly button toward the spine, flex your back foot (pointing your toes toward the ground), and keep the back of your neck long. Stay for 5-10 breaths on each side.

9. Tabletop Variation

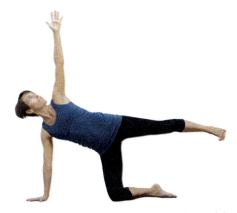

Now that you've created more strength in the hamstrings, it's time to train the sides of the hips. You'll also continue to build strength in the upper body by holding up your weight in this Tabletop Variation.

Swing your left shin back behind you for stability and press your left hand into the floor. Raise your right arm up. Then lift the right leg and turn your foot toward the side of your mat. With as little movement as possible, swing your right leg forward and back in space. Continue for 30-60 seconds before moving on to the second side.

Take Child's Pose or Downward-Facing Dog for 1 minute before moving on.

9. Standing Balance Poses

Come to stand at the front of your mat to begin this standing sequence. You'll repeat 6-7 poses on one side before completing the entire sequence on the other, increasing your body's strength and coordination. Translation—better balance and efficiency for your golf swing.

9A. Start in Mountain Pose

9B. Chair Pose
Exhale to sink your hips downward. Inhale to lift your chest.

9C. Toe Taps and Knee-To-Chest
As you inhale, shift weight to your right foot, and tap your left toes behind you. Exhale and draw your left knee into your chest. Repeat 5-10 times.

9D. Crescent Lunge Variation
Inhale to step your left foot back into Crescent Lunge. Once you have your balance, take a side stretch for 5 cycles of breath.

9E. Warrior 2
Strengthen the right outer hip even more while simultaneously opening up the right inner groin. Drop the outer edge of your back foot to the ground and open your hips and torso to the side of your mat. Hold for 5 rounds of breath.

9F. Reverse Warrior
Keep your lower body as it is and inhale to change arm positions—reach your right arm up as your left rests lightly on your left back leg. Breathe deeply for 5 rounds.

9G. Five-Pointed Star Pose
Turn all ten toes to the side of your mat. Inhale and reach your arms up.

9H. Wide-Leg Forward Fold
Exhale to fold forward. Keep your feet pressing firmly into the ground and draw the shoulder blades away from your ears. Place blocks under your hands or bend your knees if the floor is too far away. You will elongate the entire back of the body as you hold for 5-10 cycles of breath.

9I. Skater Pose
Build more stamina in the legs by moving side-to-side 5-10 times. Pause in the center before lifting your torso upright again.

9J. Pyramid Pose Preparation
This pose is excellent for maintaining a healthy, strong, and supple spine. Turn your right foot to face the front of your mat. The left foot will also turn forward slightly so your hips can square to the short edge of your mat. Inhale to lengthen the spine, keeping your hands on your hips. Exhale to fold forward. Use blocks under your hands to stay in this pose for 5 cycles of breath.

9K. Revolved Triangle Pose
Not only will you sustain a strong core, but you'll increase your twisting capacity in this posture. Place your left hand on your shin, a block, or the floor. Take your right hand to the back of your pelvis to ensure it remains level. Exhale and twist your chest to the right. Keep your right hand where it is or reach up. Hold the Revolved Triangle for 5-10 breaths.

Return to Mountain Pose (9A) when done. Pause for 1 minute between sides to observe new sensations in the body. Then, repeat the standing sequence on the other side.

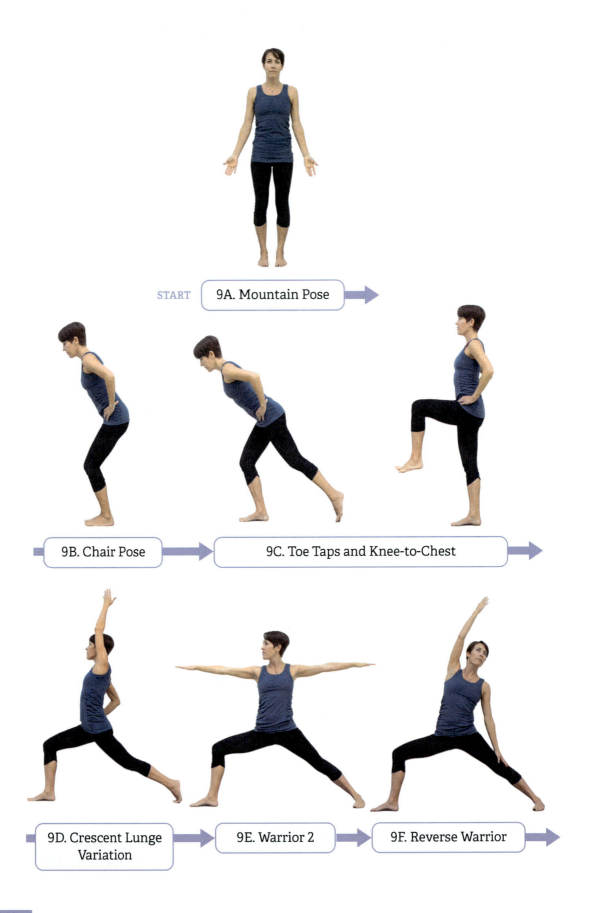

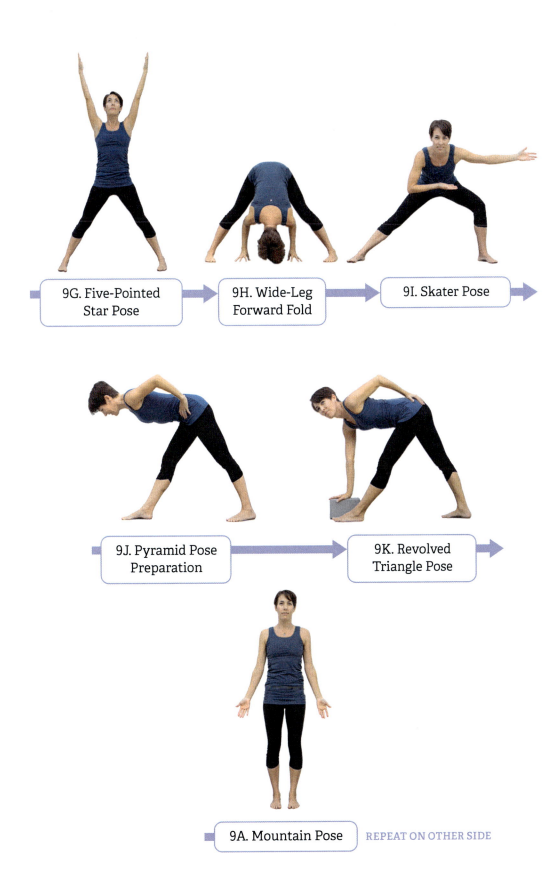

STAY GOLF-READY ALL YEAR LONG

10. Eagle Pose

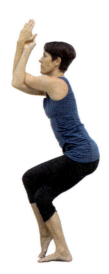

Start in Mountain Pose (Tadasana). Bend your knees slightly and cross your left thigh over the right. Point your left toes toward the floor. They can rest on the ground or hover just above it. They might even tuck behind the lower right calf. Press the right foot evenly into the floor and hug the inner thighs together.

Then, with a stable base, reach your arms out in front of you. Cross the right elbow above the left, reaching your hands to the opposite shoulders. It's like giving yourself a hug. You can stay in this position to stretch the muscles between the shoulder blades. Or, raise the forearms perpendicular to the floor with the backs of each hand facing each other. Stay here, or draw the palms closer to the midline so the palms touch (instead of the backs of the hands). Whichever expression you embody now, lift your elbows away from the floor and stretch your fingers toward the ceiling. Hold for 8 cycles of breath before switching to the other side.

11. Staff Pose

Transition from the standing poses of this sequence to the seated ones with Staff Pose.

Keep the sitting bones grounded, spine long, and heart open as your torso remains upright. See page 124 for additional notes. Breathe here for 1 minute.

12. Seated Twist

This active Seated Twist is the same pose we used in the Gentle Yoga practice on page 125. In this cross-training sequence, the pose stretches the outer hips, glutes, and hamstrings—all of which have worked throughout the class so far. Remember to sit as tall as possible as you twist toward your bent knee. Hold the pose for 10 cycles of breath.

13. Half-Cow Face Pose Variation

Continue to stretch your hamstrings and outer hips with this Half Cow Face Pose Variation. Stay upright or fold forward, keeping your spine as elongated as possible. See page 125 for more details. Breathe deeply here for 1-2 minutes.

14. Bridge Pose

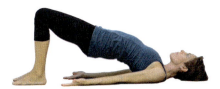

Bridge Pose is an excellent way to learn good pelvic and spinal control. The tendency here is to tighten the glutes as you lift the hips. Instead, draw the sitting bones toward the knees and imagine moving the knees forward in space. All the while, your core will keep working as you lift the hips and chest. You can also roll the shoulder blades closer together to add more depth to the pose. Hold for 5 breaths.

To come out safely, unroll the shoulders and roll the spine down one vertebra at a time. Pause for one full breath, then return to bridge pose. Complete 3 rounds of Bridge Pose before moving on to the next posture.

15. Reclined Hamstring Stretch

You used this Reclined Hamstring Stretch to restore the body after a round of golf (see page 129). Now you'll use it here to calm the body after building heat on your yoga mat. Stay for 10 cycles of breath on each side.

16. Reclined Spinal Twist

Let's take the same Reclined Spinal Twist from earlier in the sequence (see page 153). The best part about doing this at the end of class—other than it releases any remaining tension in the hips, spine, and shoulders—is that you get a clear picture of what's changed in your body as a result of your practice. Deeply relax here as you take an inventory of your entire body. Hold for 2-3 minutes on each side.

17. Final Relaxation

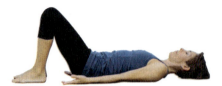

Absorb all the changes from your cross-training practice in this final resting pose (also known as Savasana). You can assume Constructive Rest Pose with the knees bent (pictured above), which can be helpful if you have any tension in the lower back. Or, extend your entire body flat on the floor as shown on page 132. Breathe naturally. Relax your muscles. Chill out as best you can while you rest in stillness. Stay for 5-10 minutes.

Activity: Cross-Training with Chair Yoga

A chair is used as a prop in this sequence to make many yoga postures more accessible. Just like the previous class, we'll use a variety of poses to activate the entire body and address golf-specific movements as well.

Time: 60 minutes
Suggested Props: A chair, a strap

1. Seated Breathing

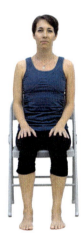

Utilize the first few minutes in a seated position to shift your focus from your day to the present moment. Close your eyes. Keep your spine long and shoulders relaxed. Observe the natural rhythm of your breathing. Notice how long it takes to breathe in and out, without trying to change it in any way. After a minute or two, consciously change the pattern of your breathing. Match the length of your inhale with that of your exhale. Keep breathing through the nose as you do this. The goal is to sustain this even breathing for the rest of the practice.

2. Cat Pose / Cow Pose

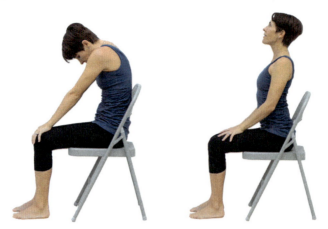

The Cat-Cow sequence is a foundational yoga move to warm up the spine. On your inhale, broaden the collarbones as you sit upright. As you exhale, reach your hands toward your knees as you round the spine. Lightly tuck your tailbone and chin into Cat Pose. On the following inhale, tilt the pelvis forward and arch the back. Roll your shoulders back and lift your gaze. This is Cow Pose. Repeat this Cat-Cow sequence five times, moving slowly with your breath. Return to a neutral spine when you're done.

3. Seated Forward Fold

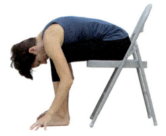

This Seated Forward Fold elongates the entire back of the body. Inhale to lengthen your spine in your seated position. Exhale and walk your hands and torso forward into a fold. You can stop with your hands or elbows on your thighs. You can go deeper and eventually have your torso and thighs meet. Relax your head and neck as much as possible once you find a 60-80% stretch in this pose. Continue to press the floor away with your feet. Stay in the fold for 5-8 cycles of breath. Then, use your inhale to roll the spine back up to a vertical position.

4. Lateral Bend

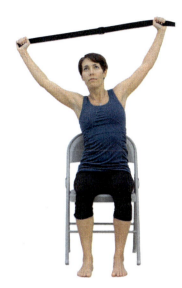

Grab your strap for this Lateral Bend. Make sure your arms are wider than your shoulders, and your palms face down as you hold the strap. The wider your grip, the easier this pose will be on your shoulders. On an inhale, reach both arms toward the ceiling as you keep the strap taut. As you exhale, reach your torso and arms over to the left. Inhale to return upright and exhale to the right. Repeat these movements 3-5 times. On the last round, hold the lateral bend for 5 rounds of breath. With your exhale, release your arms back to your lap. Place the strap on the floor before moving on.

4. Opposite Arm and Leg Extension

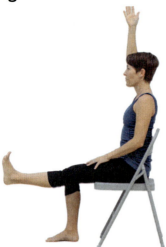

This is a seated version of Bird Dog Pose. Since it involves both sides of the body moving in opposition, communication improves between the brain's right and left hemispheres. Your core, hip flexors, and shoulders engage as well.

As you inhale, reach your right leg forward and your left arm forward. The left arm can stay parallel to the floor, or it can extend vertically toward the ceiling. As you exhale, return both limbs to your starting position at the same time. Repeat the same movements, lifting the left leg and right arm. Then complete 5 more rounds on each side.

5. Downward-Facing Dog, Variation

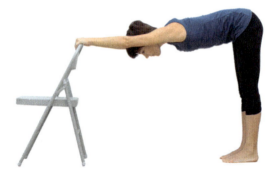

This Down Dog Variation is common in many chair classes, and it's one you used on the golf course to stay mobile. See page 107 for details. Hold for 8 cycles of breath.

6. Chair Pose

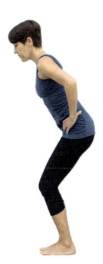

Stand next to your chair and use it for balance if needed. With your feet hip width apart, press evenly into both feet as you drop your hips down. Lift the torso upright and draw your front ribs in. Lift the arms up. Hold Chair Pose for 5 cycles of breath.

7. Toe Taps and Knee-To-Chest

Take 5-8 rounds of the Toe Tap and Knee-To-Chest exercise on page 77.

8. Warrior 2

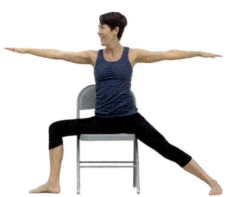

This pose can be done in a standing position, as on page (see inset page), or you can return to your chair and take Warrior 2 with support.

In this latter version, move your right leg out to the side, toes pointing 90-degrees to the right. Your hips and torso will continue to face the front of your chair. If you already notice a stretch in the inner right thigh, you can stay in this modified position. If you're ready to move on, extend the left leg out to the side. The left toes will turn inward slightly, and the left inner arch lines up with the right heel. The front ribs stay in as the lower belly lifts. Arms can stay on your hips or reach out over the legs, parallel to the floor. Hold for 8 cycles of breath. First, exhale to release your arms and reverse your steps to get out of the pose. Repeat on the left side.

9. Wide-Legged Forward Fold

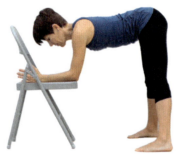

You have two options for this Wide-Legged Forward Fold. You can sit on the front edge of your chair, take your legs wide, and fold forward. Or, take this pose from a standing position. In the latter option, stand and face your chair. Place your feet 3-4 ft. apart and point all ten toes forward (or slightly inward). Inhale to lengthen the spine. As you exhale, fold the torso forward. You can use the back or seat of the chair for support. Just make sure you move the shoulder blades down the back and away from the ears as you fold. Hold for 5-8 cycles of breath before inhaling to stand once again.

10. Wide-Legged Twist

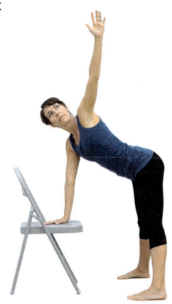

The base of this Wide-Legged Twist is the same as the pose above. Keep your feet wider than hip-distance apart and your feet pointing in the same direction as your torso. Engage the core slightly as you fold halfway forward. Place your left palm into the seat of the chair. Keep your torso parallel to the floor and start to rotate your spine to the right. You can place your right palm on your sacrum or reach the right arm up toward the sky. Continue to press down with your left hand to help you rotate. Stay for 5 cycles of breath, then use your exhale to unwind. Repeat the same pose on the other side.

11. Seated Eagle Pose

The previous two poses elongated the muscles of the inner thigh. Now, it's time to engage them in Eagle Pose. The actions will be the same as the standing version of this pose (see page 160). However, you will have more support with a chair beneath you. Hold for 8 cycles of breath on each side.

12. Seated Figure-4 Pose

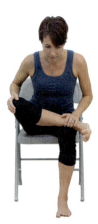

A Seated Figure-4 Pose stretches the glutes and piriformis—a small, deep hip muscle that can become inflamed when your hips are tight. Start in a seated position, with your knees over the ankles and feet hip distance apart. Press the left foot firmly into the ground. Cross your right ankle over your left knee and keep your right foot flexed. Ideally, this will be just above the right ankle and left knee, so you avoid bone-on-bone contact. Allow your right knee to drop down. Stay in this position with your spine upright if you already notice a stretch in the outer right hip. To go deeper, start to fold forward. Once you find a 60-80% stretch, stay and breathe deeply. Hold for 8-10 rounds before switching sides.

13. Seated Twist

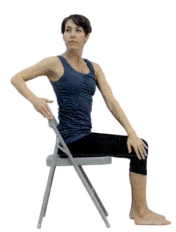

This Seated Twist will create space between each vertebra of the spine, creating more mobility as you move through everyday life and as you swing a club on the course.

Inhale and elongate your spine. Exhale and take your right hand across your left knee, and your left hand behind you on the chair. Your right shoulder blade moves away from the spine, and the left draws closer to it. Take 5 cycles of breath. Then, inhale to return to center and repeat on the other side.

14. Seated Forward Fold

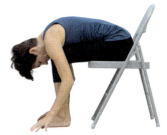

In addition to lengthening the spine, a Seated Forward Fold also becomes a mild inversion as the head moves below the heart. Use this symmetrical pose to turn your attention inward. Breathe deeply. Relax the body as much as possible. Notice the sensations in your body as you take this pose for the second time—I guarantee there will be differences! After 5-8 cycles of breath, use the inhale to sit tall once again.

15. Final Relaxation

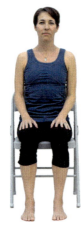
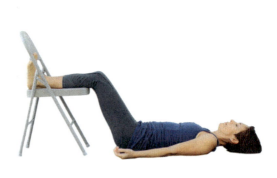

You can sit in your chair or recline on the floor for your final resting pose. The purpose is to find a position in which your body can be completely comfortable. This way, you absorb the changes of your practice and give the mind space for insight. Even if you remain seated, imagine yourself doing nothing. Relax the feet, legs, and hips. Let the shoulders drop down away from the ears. Soften your closed eyes, jaw, and throat. Breathe effortlessly for 3-5 minutes. You can even set a timer if that allows you to be more present in this last portion of your yoga practice.

Cross-Training for the Mind

Yoga puts the body in motion to train the mind into the present moment. Here is another of my favorite tools to accomplish this—one that is a wonderful resource to use between rounds. It's meditation.

Meditation is a technique in which you relax the body while keeping the mind alert. As you do this, you train the mind into the present moment. Said another way, meditation trains you to focus.

In the Tibetan language, *"to meditate"* means *"to become familiar with."* When you meditate, you turn your attention inward and become familiar with your habits. You notice when your brain is in a beta state, with thoughts bouncing frantically from the past to the future.[6]

With the eyes closed in meditation, you minimize external distractions and you start to slow down your brain wave patterns. You can travel from high beta to low beta, and into an even slower alpha state. You also start to downregulate the nervous system, which helps your body unwind.

Subtle sensations become more vibrant in this quiet space. You become more aware of your breathing, your heartbeat, and your inner wisdom (all of which get overlooked in the busyness of everyday life). This is when answers appear, and seeds of inspired action are sewn.

Scientific research confirms a meditation practice can benefit you in many ways.[7] Meditation:

- Improves physical health
- Boosts creativity
- Increases your connection with others
- Enhances self-trust
- Improves mental clarity and focus
- Leads to higher energy levels
- Reduces stress
- Enhances satisfaction with life as a whole

> *"Competitive golf is played mainly on the five-and-a-half-inch course: the space between your ears."*
>
> –Bobby Jones, professional golfer

Like yoga, meditation is a practice. Start with a simple technique, and then add more complexity as your skill set increases. And, you can add it easily into your cross-training schedule when you have the time to learn something new. Find the techniques that work for you, and blend those into your pre-season and competitive golf seasons when you're ready.

Here's another example of what your schedule might look like during your time off.

OFF-SEASON SCHEDULE WITH MEDITATION

SUNDAY OFF	MONDAY EASY	TUESDAY HARD	WEDNESDAY EASY	THURSDAY MODERATE	FRIDAY HARD	SATURDAY EASY
Morning meditation	Morning meditation	Morning meditation	Morning meditation	Morning meditation	Morning meditation	Morning meditation
Off	Moderate activity	Cross-training yoga	Walk	Off	Cross-training yoga	Off
5-min evening journal	5-min evening journal	5-min evening journal	5-min evening journal	5-min evening journal	5-min evening journal	5-min evening journal

Activity: Start a Meditation Practice

This is a short exercise to begin a meditation practice of your own. I suggest starting with 5 minutes of stillness and working your way to longer increments as you're ready.

Step 1: Find a Quiet Place
The goal is to be undisturbed while you meditate, so turn off your phone and select a space where you won't be interrupted by others.

Step 2: Establish a Focal Point
The goal of meditation is to train the mind into the present moment. You'll select a focal point to help with this process. You can choose:
- An image, like your ball flying high in the sky toward the hole as your body is relaxed
- The count of your breathing (like what we did in week 3)
- The heartbeat in your chest (as a sound or sensation)
- The hum of the HVAC unit or your refrigerator
- Sensations on your skin

Now close your eyes and keep your attention on your selected point of focus.

Step 3: Bring Your Attention Back
Your mind will likely wander, despite your intention to stay focused. Each time you notice your thoughts wander from your focal point, take a deeper breath. Inwardly smile as if you were training an adorable puppy. Then, return your inner gaze to your focal point.

Step 4: Notice any Changes
When your timer goes off, take another deep round of breath. Then, slowly open your eyes and pay attention to the space around you once again. Notice any changes in the mind or body as a result of your time in stillness.

Avoid These Cross-Training Pitfalls

Yes, I encourage you to use yoga between rounds to boost your health and well-being. However, there are pitfalls you can avoid when doing so to get the most out of your time on the mat.

Trying Too Hard

Yoga is not your sport—golf is. So, don't go too hard, too fast when you hit the yoga mat. Explore an intensity level your body can meet consistently.

Too Much Duration

Duration refers to the amount of time you spend on an activity. With yoga, you want to begin with shorter classes first. Then, you can add more time as your stamina increases.

Practicing Too Frequently

Frequency refers to how many days each week you practice yoga. One day per week will help you keep your current flexibility level; practicing at least two will help you make gains. It's also true that the more you practice something, the better you get at it, and the quicker your body adjusts. Start with fewer classes at the beginning, and check-in with your energy levels often. You can then adjust how often you practice yoga as is suitable for your body and schedule.

Practicing Too Soon After a Round

Remember, the body has lower energy levels within the 24-48 hours after play. During this period, a restorative focus or slower active recovery yoga class is best. Then you can amplify the intensity as you enter the supercompensation phase.

Putting it Together

A yoga cross-training plan keeps your positive momentum going between rounds. It also provides a structure in which you can maximize the elements of a golf-ready body. You stay stronger and more mobile. Your mind is more alert. And each time you step on your yoga mat, you generate more energy to use on the course for many healthy years to come. The trick is to start simple and honor your goals as you practice.

Take Action Now

- **Review your intentions as a golfer.**
  Ask yourself who you want to be as a golfer and what you want to accomplish. You can also revisit the Flexible Golfer Questionnaire on page 23 to gain more clarity.

- **Practice yoga.**
  Unroll your yoga mat and give the chair or floor-based yoga class a try this week. You guessed it! I'll lead you through each pose at TheFlexibleGolfer.com/free

- **Create a yoga cross-training plan.**
  Use your new knowledge to create a program that matches your current schedule, fitness level, and intentions. You can add one cross-training tool for the body or mind at first. Then add on as your time and energy allow.

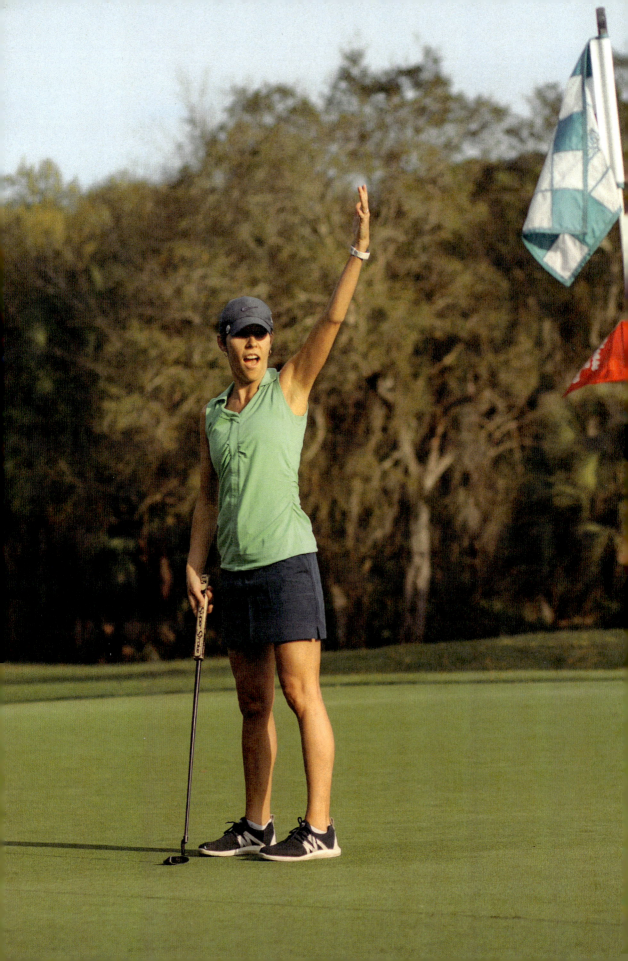

CONCLUSION

Putting it Together

"What you know matters little if you don't put it into practice."
–Todd Henry

OVERVIEW

Endings are a reason to celebrate because you can savor your progress. You get to blend your passion for golf and new knowledge of yoga into meaningful actions that move you closer to your goals. And, you can springboard from this inspiration into new beginnings ahead. We'll tap into this, and more, in our last moments here together.

Pull up a chair and let's chat for a few minutes. You have done an incredible job learning about yoga over the past six weeks. You've applied concepts in fresh ways and put these techniques to the test with your body and mind. This takes courage and dedication. I'm so proud of you!

I liken what you've just accomplished to taking a drink of water from a bursting fire hydrant.

It might seem astonishing. Dare I say, a bit overwhelming.

That's why I want to recap what just happened. The goal with this is threefold.

First, I want us to acknowledge the sheer amount of information you just inhaled. You have wired your brain in new ways and you are ready to embrace a new you, a new golf game, a new future.

Second, I want this information to stick around. I want these neural networks to keep firing in your brain so they become second nature. This involves a review of the material. It also requires you to revisit it continually.

Finally, I want to reinforce that these ideas are simpler than you think. You likely incorporate several of these ingredients into your life already. We're just going to highlight why the techniques work, and how you might tweak them in ways that are most enjoyable and realistic for your life.

The easiest way to accomplish this is with the simple table below. In the left-hand column, we have each method you learned in this book. Then in the right-hand column, you'll discover when and why to apply these tools for maximum benefit.

METHOD/TOOL	WHY AND WHEN TO USE IT
Brain-Integrated Posture	This crossover pattern reduces stress, boosts creativity, and makes it easier to learn, and recall, information. Use it when you're flustered or anxious. Or sit in this pose before learning something new to create a superlearning state.
Breathing, Awareness of	Paying attention to your breathing returns your focus to the present moment, giving you more control, awareness, and clarity.
Breathing, Box	Match the length of the inhale with the length of the exhale to establish equanimity in the body and mind.
Breathing, Exhale-focused	Create a longer outbreath than inbreath to stimulate the relaxation response in the body. This works wonders when you are overstimulated before or after golf.
Breathing, Inhale-focused	Make your inhale longer than your exhale to stimulate or energize your system. Use this if you are tired or sluggish.
Comfort Kit	This is a logistical care kit of items you put together before a round of golf to ensure your needs are met on the course.
Corpse Pose (Final Relaxation)	Also known as Savasana, this reclined posture is taken at the end of a yoga class to integrate changes made on the mat. You can also lie on your back and breathe consciously to relax and return balance to the body and mind.
Cross-Training, Yoga	Cross-training yoga classes incorporate a variety of styles and movements to generate more strength, balance, mobility, and coordination. These enhance your golf swing and your ability to function in everyday life.
Dristi (gazing point)	Select a relevant focal point to increase concentration when it's needed in your golf game. Then, shift your gaze away from your game to anything on the course to stay present, conserving energy during your round. It also opens your mind up to greater possibilities during play.

METHOD/TOOL	WHY AND WHEN TO USE IT
Dynamic Stretching	This active style of yoga moves your joints through a full range of motion and is best used before golf to prepare you for the powerful golf swing. It also helps prevent injuries. We use dynamic stretching in cross-training yoga classes as a way to warm-up the body as well.
Eyes Closed	By closing your eyes, you decrease the stimuli from your environment and start to downregulate the nervous system. You can pair breathing, visualization, or meditation techniques with your eyes closed to amplify the power of those processes as well. This can be done on the course or any time in your day you want to regroup, gain control, or have greater insight about a decision.
Flex the Muscles of Your Mind	This activity transforms the negative dialogue of your mind into positive, constructive speech that supports your game. I suggest using it between rounds of golf to identify any inner blocks. Then, you can remove those hindrances and regroup before you play again. The end result is you're internally aligned before taking action. And you bridge the gap between where you are now and where you want to go in the future.
Gentle Yoga	Slow, deliberate movements in this style of yoga increase circulation, reduce stiffness, and counteract inflammation. This is best used after a round of golf or between rounds when your body is slow or fatigued.
Gratitude Journal	When you focus on positive emotions, like gratitude and appreciation, you create heart coherence. This translates to a release of life-enhancing chemicals in the body, increased cognitive function, and more mental clarity.
Intention, Set an	An intention clarifies what you want. You can use it before a round, before a single shot, or before your entire season to more deeply understand yourself and the best path forward.

METHOD/TOOL	WHY AND WHEN TO USE IT
Mantra (word or phrase)	Ward off unwanted distractions and sustain concentration on your game by repeating a meaningful word or phrase on the golf course.
Meditation	Meditation is a technique that trains the mind to relax while the body remains alert. You shift your focus inward, change your brain wave patterns, and relax into the present moment. This is a great tool to use between rounds of golf to improve focus, trust your swing, and sustain higher levels of energy.
Myofascial Release (MFR)	MFR techniques manipulate your muscles and fascia through compression or rolling. You can use them to release tension in the body and combat repetitive movements that cause imbalance.
Point-and-Call	Increase your focus on the golf course by identifying and verbalizing the important elements of the moment. This acts as a verbal cue to boost your awareness.
Pre-Shot Routine (PIVOT)	This 5-part plan helps your body and mind work together before each hit you take on the golf course.
Props, Yoga	In addition to your yoga mat, you can use blocks, blankets, bolsters, and straps to support your practice. These props make it easier to get into various poses on your yoga mat. They also keep your body safe as you learn different postures.

REST Formula	Recovery after your round of golf requires relaxation, and the REST formula reminds you of each ingredient to restore overall balance.
	    R = Resilience for the body (yoga, massage, etc.)
	    E = Equanimity of mind (breathing, meditation)
	    S = Self-Study (reflection)
	    T = Time-Saving Actions (organization/cleaning)

METHOD/TOOL	WHY AND WHEN TO USE IT
Restorative Yoga	This style of yoga uses longer, supported holds to downregulate the nervous system. It's excellent to incorporate after a round of golf or anytime in life you are overly stressed.
Static Stretching	Static stretching is both active and passive. We engage parts of the body to lengthen others in active static stretches. We use short holds before golf and longer ones in yoga cross-training classes. Then we use passive static stretching in Yin and Restorative Yoga.
Subtle Activation	In week 1, you learned how to activate the feet, stabilize the hips, engage the core, and mobilize the shoulders. These simple activities turn on the muscles in subtle ways that prepare you for the powerful golf swing. I suggest you use these exercises between rounds to enhance the awareness and communication in your entire body.
Visualization	Any time you want to create a future memory or picture the best event occurring in your round (or with your shot), engage your imagination. See what you want to have happen. Then mentally rehearse what you would hear and feel as well. This trains the subconscious mind to expect a new outcome.
Yin Yoga	Yin Yoga uses longer holds to target the ligaments, tendons, and fascia. Little energy is required, so it's best used after golf. Or you can incorporate it between rounds for long-term shifts in your range of motion.

How to Best Move Forward

I understand there is not a one-size-fits-all approach to achieving your golf goals. Different strategies work for different people. This is why I provide a number of techniques throughout this book. It is also why I want to address the topic of motivation now.

Motivation is the driving force that inspires you to implement these strategies. It's the processes you use to pursue, and ultimately embody, your desires.

You have so many yoga tools in your yoga toolbox now! As you stay motivated, you can frequently put them into action to improve your golf game, up-level your health, and mitigate injuries.

Your capacity to do this revolves around two things: [1]

- Expectations you have for yourself (self-imposed ideas, like practicing on the range 3 times per week this summer)
- Expectations others have for you (pressures placed on you by outside forces, like teammates expecting you to play well during a tournament)

If you naturally like to meet inner and outer expectations, you've likely planned how to integrate yoga into your golf routine already. Way to go! I admire your go-get 'em attitude and dedication to taking action. Keep in mind that as you blend your intuition and common sense, you'll stay more energized as you apply these new tools.

If you're motivated internally but still not sure about the long-term benefits of yoga to your golf game, you'll likely do more research. This is exactly why I have an extensive index for you to learn more about the various topics in this book. I suggest you keep learning while you implement this knowledge to avoid analysis paralysis. And, I must say, I find your curiosity contagious. Keep it up! This attribute can be your superpower on the course (and in life).

You might notice you're more likely to prioritize the expectations of others over your own. You definitely show up when someone is counting on you. I deeply appreciate how this makes you reliable and dedicated. Let's use the momentum of these gifts to stick with your yoga practice, too. I recommend you grab a yoga buddy or enlist other members of your club to join you on the yoga mat. Maybe even have your spouse dangle the carrot of a new golf bag as a reward for sticking with your program. Just remember that saying *"Yes"* to fewer, but meaningful, yoga commitments can make your progress more enjoyable.

If you consider yourself a rebel, and like to do things your own way in your own time, use this to your advantage as you blend yoga into your golf-loving life. Don't bind yourself to a particular routine. Try new styles of yoga and regularly mix up your approach. I know that you will find a way that works for you, and I applaud the ingenuity you bring to the table.

Regardless of the intentions you have for yourself or the expectations others have of you, no matter your age, fitness level, current life responsibilities, or hours spent on the golf course each week, there is one thing I know to be true. You're at your best when the body and mind work as one. You can achieve incredible heights when you step just beyond your comfort zone and take action with confident ease.

The power to do this is already within you. This harmony you seek is your birthright.

You now have the awareness and tools to tap into this infinite reservoir regularly. And I believe you will do so incredibly well on your journey forward as a flexible golfer.

Next Steps

Visit TheFlexibleGolfer.com/free for:

Worksheets
I created a set of printable worksheets to help you apply the principles in this book in a practical way. They'll also keep you focused as you progress toward your golf, and life, goals.

Yoga Classes
Skip the guesswork about each pose and join me on the yoga mat as I lead you through each yoga sequence in this book.

Start Fresh Sundays
This is a short weekly email designed to encourage and inspire you on your journey. Plus, I share the latest scientific research and practice tips to uplevel your game.

Group Resources and Materials
If you'd like to study The Flexible Golfer with your golf club, we have question prompts and suggested best practices to explore, and implement, the weekly material in a group setting.

Visit TheFlexibleGolfer.com for:

Events and Workshops
Let me help you unlock your potential, tap into more strength, and stay golf-ready with our in-person and virtual events.

Acknowledgements

Authors speak of writing as a solitary journey, yet this book is nothing short of a collaborative miracle. A huge thank you to my honest and detail-oriented editor, Krista Wenz, who pushed the bounds of time to refine this text. I deeply appreciate my talented photographers, Diane Clifford and Jina Morgese. You ladies see beyond the obvious and capture the magnificent. To Danielle Alling—a bright light who entered my world just over a year ago. You listen carefully, generously sprinkle in your creative genius, and transform the gazillion ideas in my head into a cohesive, beautiful masterpiece.

If home is where your heart is, then mine is forever with Kevin, Ronnie, and the entire Bailey Creek crew. Together you craft the most beautiful and welcoming golf course I know. This is also true of the Bailey Creek women's club. Massive thanks to each adventurous, vibrant, and kind member. You taught me well in the ways of golf and continue to amplify my enjoyment of the game each summer.

To the amazing team at Buttermilk, who fed my soul and belly during this entire writing process.

To my family by blood, the growing Coco and Hahn clan, whose playfulness and unconditional love inspire me to shine bright. To my family by choice—Marilyn, Rachel, Christina, Bobbie, and Robin—for encouraging me to reach higher. To my husband and soulmate, Steve, for his unwavering support. And to Kai, my stubborn Staffy, who reminds me to get outside and mix things up daily.

The light in me bows to the light in each of you. Namaste!

Resources

The following is a partial list of the scientific articles, books, and online resources you can utilize should you want to learn more about any idea or concept expressed in this book. This is not an exhaustive list, but it will open doors for further research and inquiry.

This Thing Called Yoga

1. Dr. Craig Davies and Vince DiSaia, *Golf Anatomy* (Champaign, Illinois: Human Kinetics, 2019).
2. Sengupta, P. "Health Impacts of Yoga and Pranayama: A State-of-the-Art Review." *Int J Prev Med*. 3, 1. (Jul 2012): 444–458.
3. Chris Crowley and Henry Lodge, *Younger Next Year: Live Strong, Fit, and Sexy—Until You're 80 and Beyond* (New York; Workman Publications, 2004).
4. Dr. Joe Dispenza, *Breaking the Habit of Being Yourself* (Carlsbad, California: Hay House, Inc, 2012).
5. Steven Kotler and Jamie Wheal, *Stealing Fire* (New York: Dey St, 2017).
6. Mihaly Csikszentmihalyi, *Flow: The Psychology of Optimal Experience* (New York: HarperCollins, 1990).
7. Sri Swami Satchidananda, *The Yoga Sutras of Patanjali* (Buckingham, Virginia: Integral Yoga Publications, 1978).
8. TKV Desikachar, *The Heart of Yoga* (Rochester, Vermont: Inner Traditions International, 1995).
9. James Clear, *Atomic Habits* (New York: Avery, 2018).
10. https://www.manduka.com

Week 1: Explore the Golf-Body in Motion

1. Bob Rotella, *Golf is Not a Game of Perfect* (New York: Simon and Schuster, 2007).
2. Dr. Craig Davies and Vince DiSaia, *Golf Anatomy* (Champaign, Illinois: Human Kinetics, 2019).
3. Leslie Kaminoff and Amy Matthews, *Yoga Anatomy* (Champaign, Illinois: Human Kinetics, 2007).

Week 2: Flex the Muscles of your Mind

1. Dr. Norman Doidge, *The Brain that Changes Itself* (New York: Penguin Books, 2007).
2. Dr. Joe Dispenza, *Breaking the Habit of Being Yourself* (Carlsbad, California: Hay House, Inc, 2012).
3. Dr. Joe Dispenza, *Evolve your Brain: The Science of Changing your Mind* (Carlsbad, California: Hay House, Inc, 2012).
4. R. Douglas Fields, *Electric Brain* (Dallas, Texas: Benbella Books, 2020).
5. Robert M. Sapolsky, *Why Zebras Don't Get Ulcers* (New York: Henry Holt and Company, 2004).
6. Candace Pert, PhD, *Molecules of Emotion* (New York: Touchstone, 1997).
7. Bessel van der Kolk M.D., *The Body Keeps the Score* (New York: Penguin Books, 2015).
8. Bruce Lipton, PhD, *The Biology of Belief* (Carlsbad, California: Hay House, Inc, 2008).
9. HeartMath Institute. (2021, March 15) *Science of the Heart: Exploring the Role of the Heart in Human Performance.* https://www.heartmath.org/research/science-of-the-heart/
10. Todd Herman, *The Alter Ego Effect: The Power of Secret Identities to Transform Your Life* (New York: HarperCollins, 2019).

Week 3: Develop a Pre-Round Routine

1. Dr. Craig Davies and Vince DiSaia, *Golf Anatomy* (Champaign, Illinois: Human Kinetics, 2019).
2. Peck, Evan MD, Greg Chomko DPT, Dan Gaz V. MS, and Ann M. Farrell MLS. "The Effects of Stretching on Performance." *Current Sports Medicine Reports.* 13, 3 (May/June 2014): 179-185.
3. Behm, D.G. and A Chaouachi. "A review of the acute effects of static and dynamic stretching on performance." *Eur J Appl Physiol.* 111 (2011): 2633–2651.
4. Opplert, J. and N. Babault. "Acute Effects of Dynamic Stretching on Muscle Flexibility and Performance: An Analysis of the Current Literature." *Sports Med.* 48 (2018): 299–325.
5. Lin, WC, CL Lee, and NJ Chang. "Acute Effects of Dynamic Stretching Followed by Vibration Foam Rolling on Sports Performance of Badminton Athletes." *J Sports Sci Med.* 19, 2 (2020): 420-428.
6. Yue, G. and KJ Cole. "Strength Increases from the Motor Program: Comparison of Training with Maximal Voluntary and Imagined Muscle Contractions." *J Neurophysiol.* 67, 5 (May 1992): 1114-23.

7. Ranganathan, VK, V Siemionow, JZ Liu, V Sahgal, and GH Yue. "From Mental Power to Muscle Power—Gaining Strength by Using the Mind." *Neuropsychologia*. 42, 7 (2004): 944-56.
8. Yao WX, VK Ranganathan, D Allexandre, V Siemionow, and GH Yue. "Kinesthetic Imagery Training of Forceful Muscle Contractions Increases Brain Signal and Muscle Strength." *Front Hum Neurosci*. 7 (2013): 561.

Week 4: Conserve Energy on the Course

1. Tim Ferriss, *Tribe of Mentors* (Boston, Massachusetts: Houghton Mifflin Harcourt, 2017).
2. "focus." Merriam-Webster.com. Merriam-Webster, 2011. Web. 20 March 2021.
3. "Scholarly Publications." *The Center for Healthy Minds,* The University of Wisconsin. https://centerhealthyminds.org/science/publications
4. Treves, I., L Tello, R Davidson, and S Goldberg. "The relationship between mindfulness and objective measures of body awareness: A meta-analysis." *Scientific Reports*. 9 (2019): 17386.
5. Gardner, F. and Z Moore. "A mindfulness-acceptance-commitment-based approach to athletic performance enhancement: Theoretical considerations." *Behavior Therapy*. 35, 4 (2004): 707-723.
6. Steven Pressfield, *The Legend of Bagger Vance* (New York: Avon Books, 1995).
7. Paul and Gail Dennison, *Brain Gym: Simple Activities for Whole Brain Learning* (Ventura, California: Edu Kinesthetics, 1992).

Week 5: Recover With a Post-Round Ritual

1. Sage Roundtree, *The Athlete's Guide to Recovery* (Boulder, Colorado: Velo Press, 2011).
2. Daniel Pink, *When: The Scientific Secrets of Perfect Timing* (New York: Riverhead Books, 2018).
3. "Fascia Research 2015—State of the Art." *Fascia Congress*. https://www.fasciacongress.org/pdfs/FasciaConferenceBook_Introduction2015.pdf
4. Søren Kierkegaard, Journalen JJ:167 (1843), Søren Kierkegaards Skrifter, (Copenhagen: Søren Kierkegaard Research Center Copenhagen, 1997), 18, 306.

Week 6: Stay Golf-Ready All Year Long
1. Gary Mack and David Casstevens, Mind Gym (New York: McGraw-Hill, 2001).
2. David G. Behm, *The Science and Physiology of Flexibility and Stretching* (New York: Routledge, 2019).
3. Wallin, D., B Ekblom, R Grahn, and T Nordenborg. "Improvement of Muscle Flexibility. A comparison between two techniques." *American Journal of Sports Medicine*. 2 (2014): 166-170.
4. Simon Sinek, *The Infinite Game* (New York: Portfolio/Penguin Books, 2019.
5. Apostolopoulos, N. Performance Flexibility. In: *High Performance Sports Conditioning*. B Foran, Ed (Champaign, Illinois: Human Kinetics, 2001).
6. We have a beginner's class in meditation called The 3H Project. Visit TheFlexibleGolfer.com/3H-Project for more information.
7. Daniel Goleman and Richard J. Davidson, *Altered Traits: Science Reveals How Meditation Changes your Mind, Brain, and Body* (New York: Avery Books, 2017).

Putting it Together
1. Gretchen Rubin, *The Four Tendencies* (New York: Harmony Books, 2017).

Additional Image Credits
Monterey golf course: Photogolfer
Human muscle anatomy: Stihii
Foot Anatomy: Aksanaku
Adbominals: MedicalStock
Shoulder Anatomy: VectorMine
Spinal Column: Udaix
Brain Waves: Artellia

Index

Abdominals *(see core)*

Awareness 7-8, 17, 25, 29, 57-59, 71, 96, 103, 136, 140, 181

Backswing 33-34, 38-39, 41, 74, 81

Balance 5-6, 25, 29, 115-116, 145, 156-159, 181, 183.

Beliefs 51-52, 54, 61-64, 100, 182

Brain 7, 9-10, 52-54, 58-61, 86, 96, 100, 117, 173, 180-181, 183

Breath 14, 22, 100-101, 105

Breathing 11, 16, 59, 62-63, 102-103, 117, 135-136, 152, 163, 175, 181,

Chair Yoga 13-14, 163

Core 7, 32, 34, 38, 184
  poses to engage 40, 77-78, 80, 82, 107, 124-125, 154-161, 165-169,
  muscles of the 36, 39

Downswing 7, 43-44

Emotions 51, 54-56, 59-60, 104, 182

Endings 113, 137-139

Energy 8-9, 16-17, 29, 33, 38, 43, 52, 57, 59-60, 70-72, 84, 90, 93-96, 113-116, 145, 149,

Fascia 10, 46, 59, 118-123, 127-128, 140, 183-184

Feet 5-7, 29-33, 43-44, 72, 123, 138-139, 184

Flexibility 4-5, 13, 25, 33-34, 41, 44, 147, 176

Focus 9, 11, 17, 58, 85-86, 95-98, 136, 173, 181-183

Follow-Through 44

Golf Warm-Up 84

Gratitude 59, 65, 182

Hips 32-34, 43-44, 184
  poses to strengthen 35, 77-80, 82, 155-161, 166
  poses to stretch 75, 81-82, 106-107, 125-126, 129-131, 153-162, 164-165, 168-171

Hydration 120-121, 134
  of body tissue 73, 118-120, 153

Hypermobility 46

Injury 46, 72, 123
  prevention of 25, 39, 41, 121, 128

Intention 85-86, 96, 104, 146, 182

Learning 18, 53, 57-59, 63, 181, 185

Logistics 18-20, 84, 87, 137-138

Mind 9-10, 15-18, 51-52, 57-58, 61-64, 93-95, 134-136, 140, 173-175, 181-184

Mantra 98-99

Mobility 4-5, 25, 33, 41, 72-73, 127, 145, 171, 181

Myofascial Release (MFR) 119, 121, 123, 127-128, 183

Nerves 16, 71, 120

Nervous system 7, 14, 53, 58, 95, 112-118, 140, 145, 173, 182, 184

Posture 38-39, 45, 127
    brain-integrated 62-64, 100, 181
Power 7-9, 25, 28, 33, 39, 43, 118, 149
Pranayama 16, 100-103, 114, 135
Pre-round 70-73
    checklist 88
    golf warm-up 84
    logistics 87
    yoga poses 74-83
Pre-shot routine 104-105, 183
Props 19-20

Recovery 112-113
    checklist 140
    phases of 113-115
    poses for 123-133
Resilience 95, 116, 118, 134, 140

Shoulder(s) 7, 32-33, 36-37, 41, 43-44, 184
    poses to strengthen 42, 78-79, 82, 106, 154-155, 160, 165-166
    poses to stretch 42, 76, 82, 106, 108, 127-129, 131, 160, 165-166
Spine 5, 16, 32-33, 38-39, 41, 43-45, 72,
    backbends for 127, 130, 161, 164
    forward folds for 75, 81, 107, 124-126, 153-154, 157m 159, 164, 166, 168, 170
    inversions of 132, 154, 161, 172
    side bends for 76, 79, 129, 156, 158, 165,

    rotation, twists of the 78, 82, 106, 125, 131, 153, 157, 159, 169, 171
Strength 7-9, 11, 13, 25, 33-34, 39, 145, 149, 181
Stress 53-54, 56, 59, 61, 112, 114, 117
Stretching, Types of 73, 114, 151

Tension 8-9, 59, 100, 116, 118, 121-123, 152, 183

Upswing *(see backswing)*
Visualization 10-11, 58, 86, 88, 105, 182, 184
Willpower 52, 56

Yoga 3, 11, 15-17
    after golf 123-133
    before golf 30, 35, 42, 74-83
    cross-training 145-146, 152-172
    gentle 118
    myths of 10-15
    on the course 106-108
    restorative 13-14, 118
    tips to start 18-22
    yin 13-14, 118

Zone, The 3, 17-18

About the Author

Kym Coco is a 500-hour certified yoga teacher and author of the book, *It Just Makes Sense: 7 Principles of a Joyful and Stress-Free Life.* After dedicating 15 years to competitive soccer, she traded in her cleats for a master's degree in sports kinesiology and a yoga mat.

This drastically shifted the way Kym approached her own training. For the past two decades, she has passed on these yoga techniques to college athletes and senior citizens alike for improved performance and injury prevention. The principles also formed the perfect foundation to excel on the course when bitten by the golf bug just a few short years ago.

Kym calls Florida home. However, she spends half of the year traveling the United States via Sprinter van sharing The Flexible Golfer program.

Made in the USA
Las Vegas, NV
28 December 2021

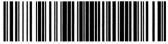